Manual of Bone
Marrow Examination

Manual of Bone Marrow Examination

Anwarul Islam, M.D., Ph.D., MRCPath

Clinical Assistant Professor of Medicine
State University of New York
at Buffalo
Attending Physician,
Buffalo General Hospital,
Buffalo, New York,
USA

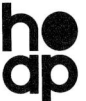

harwood academic publishers
Australia • Canada • China • France • Germany • India • Japan
Luxembourg • Malaysia • The Netherlands • Russia • Singapore
Switzerland • Thailand

1st Floor
Amsteldijk 166
1079 LH Amsterdam
The Netherlands

British Library Cataloguing in Publication Data

Islam, Anwarul
  Manual of bone marrow examination
  1. Bone marrow – Examination – Handbooks, manuals, etc.
  2. Bone marrow – Biopsy – Handbooks, manuals, etc.
  I. Title
  616.4'1'07'58

  ISBN 90-5702-009-2

Dedication

To my Parents
and to my wife Shelly
and sons Dimitri and Pierre

Contents

Contents

Preface

The purpose of this manual is to present a systematic approach to the methods of procurement and examination of bone marrow (aspiration and trephine biopsy) samples which play a crucial role in the diagnosis and management of haematological as well as non-haematological conditions. The manual is designed for medical students, house officers, physicians and other health professionals with an interest in haematology and oncology. It can also be used as a readily available, contemporary reference source for technologists and nurses who are involved in assisting in bone marrow biopsy procurement and processing of marrow for cytological, immunological and histological examination. Although most practicing haematologists are familiar with bone marrow sampling techniques for diagnostic evaluation there is a growing body of information that merits review, critical analysis and consolidation in one working reference.

The manual is organised into two major sections. The first is directed towards an appreciation of the merits, advantages, disadvantages and limitations of bone marrow aspiration biopsies. The selection of biopsy site(s) and the diagnostic value of the derived Romanowsky stained dry film smears are discussed. The second section of the text addresses the trephine or solid core bone marrow biopsy. Particular attention is directed to the new and improved instrumentation that has been introduced into the field. In addition to comparing the core biopsy with the aspiration biopsy technique the particular advantages of the former procedure are evaluated in detail. Finally, considerable attention has been given to the stepwise bedside technique of obtaining ideal bone marrow biopsy specimens and their processing.

It is recognised that bone marrow biopsy is a specialised clinical procedure. It is associated with well recognised requirements as well as potential problems that are less well known. These considerations and their resolution from a clinical haematologist's viewpoint are specifically included in this text.

Acknowledgements

I am greatly indebted to Professor Chester Glomski, M.D. for his unfailing enthusiasm and help in writing this book. I am also grateful to Paul Gliddon of Downs Surgical (UK) for providing me with some of the original illustrations. I would also like to express my sincere appreciation and thanks to Elena Greco for her excellent art work. In addition I am grateful to Harwood Academic Publishers for their constant help, interest and continued support in completing this text.

CHAPTER 1

INTRODUCTION

INTRODUCTION TO BONE MARROW AND ITS EXAMINATION

Bone marrow is housed within the inner fixed confines of bone and is the haematopoietic organ responsible for the production of the blood cellular elements that perform vital functions of oxygen transport, protection against bacterial and viral pathogens, control of inflammatory responses, and participation in endothelial repair as well as clot formation. The importance of bone marrow examination in any haematological disorder cannot be over emphasized. In its absence the investigation of any haematopoietic disorder, unless otherwise well defined, documented and prognostically evaluated, is incomplete. Even in many cases where the diagnosis is clinically and pathologically established an examination of the bone marrow remains an integral part of the practice of effective, scientific, haematologic medicine.

CYTOLOGIC AND HISTOLOGIC ANALYSIS

There are two methods available for diagnostic access to the bone marrow, cytologic and histologic. In the former approach, i.e. bone marrow aspiration, a sample of marrow is withdrawn from a bone via an aspirating needle and a syringe delivering a mixture of free haematopoietic cells, small aggregates or clusters of marrow cells and fat (often termed bone marrow particles, fragments or units), and a variable amount of sinusoidal blood. This material is itilized to prepare dry film smears which are typically stained with a Romanowsky type dye (Leishman, Giemsa etc.). Conversely in the histologic analysis of bone marrow, a biopsy is obtained which provides an undisturbed segment of marrow tissue with its cellular, vascular and osseus *in situ* relationships intact. This tissue is then fixed in a suitable fixative and prepared for paraffin or plastic embedding, sectioning, staining, and subsequent analysis.

ACCESS TO BONE MARROW

Various sites are available for the access of haematopoitic bone marrow in man. Satisfactory samples can be routinely aspirated from the sternum, the iliac crest(s) in the region of the anterior or posterior iliac spines and the spinous processes

MARROW ASPIRATION AND BIOPSY SITES

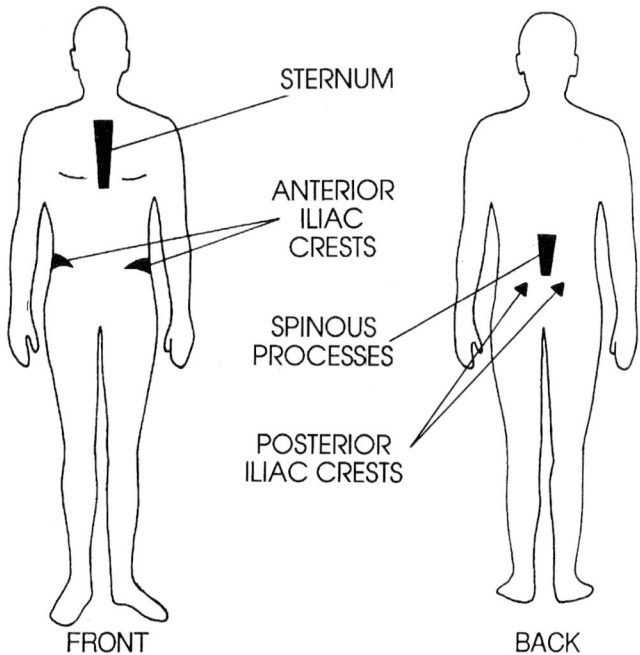

FIGURE 1. Access to bone marrow.

of the lumbar vertebrae (Figure 1). The region of the tibial proximal epiphysis is an excellent safe site for sampling in children but is not appropriate for adults because of the replacement of its red marrow with adipose cells (inactive yellow marrow). Sternal puncture has historically been the most commonly used technique of aspirating bone marrow. In recent years, however, due to the availability of improved, more durable bone marrow aspiration instruments the region of the posterior iliac spine has become more frequently the site of choice. Bone marrow histologic (solid tissue) biopsies, often termed needle or core biopsies, are usually performed at the anterior or posterior iliac crests. Again, as a result of technological improvements as well as ease of access the posterior locus is becoming more frequently utilized.

QUANTITATIVE REQUIREMENTS FOR ASPIRATION AND SECTIONED TISSUE SAMPLING

For routine bone marrow cytology the amount of marrow required to be aspirated is minimal. Usually 0.3–0.5 ml is sufficient to prepare several dry film smears.

Small volumes are also cited as advantageous because this prevents a dilution of the haematopoietic cells with circulating blood and its cellular contents. Larger volumes may be necessary when cytogenetic and and/or fluorescent flow cytometric analyses are required. For solid tissue (needle) biopsies a 15–20 millimeter-long core of marrow tissue should be obtained to insure the retrieval of adequate, histlogically representative, undisturbed specimens. Sections of variable, limited usefulness are also sometimes obtainable by collecting excess bone marrow units from an aspirate, allowing them to aggregate in a plasma/thromboplastin clot and submitting this mass to the embedding and sectioning process.

CHAPTER 2
BONE MARROW ASPIRATION

STERNAL PUNCTURE

Introduction

In 1929, Mikhail Innokent'evich Arinkin (Figure 2) a Russian physician first introduced the technique of bone marrow aspiration from the sternum when he used a lumbar puncture (spinal tap) needle to obtain a marrow aspirate from this site. Since then sternal puncture has become one of the most common intraosseus diagnostic procedures used in the field of haematology. Although the structure in adult humans which yields the largest quantity of bone marrow is the posterior ilium, the sternum has remained one of the most commonly used sites for obtaining aspirates for haematological diagnosis. This preferential selection may be due to the fact that this locus of haematopoietic marrow is near the surface of the body and is easily accessible.

Site

Sternal puncture is normally performed in the upper part of the body of the sternum, below the sternal angle of Louis and opposite the second intercostal space, midway between the midsternal line and the right or left sternal border (Figure 3). This particular site is chosen because the needle enters one of the previous centers of ossification where the red marrow is usually more abundant than in the midsternal line. The sternum is most stable at this level and least likely to move or fracture under applied pressure. This area is also separated from the underlying great vessels by a distance of 2–3 cm, while at the levels of third and fourth intercostal spaces, the sternum lies in close proximity to the pericardium and heart.

The manubrium of the sternum can also be used as a site for obtaining bone marrow aspirates and is perhaps the safest area of this bone to puncture. But as a rule, particularly in elderly subjects, the manubrium contains more adipose cells than the sternal body and as a result an aspiration at this site may yield an inadequate or non-representative marrow sample. However, completely satisfactory samples are obtained more often than not from the manubrium. If the manubrium is selected for aspiration, the appropriate site for the puncture is about 1 cm above the sterno-manubrial angle and slightly lateral to the mid-line.

Instrumentation

The needles most commonly used for obtaining bone marrow aspirate samples from the sternum are the Salah and Klima needles (Figure 4) or their modifications.

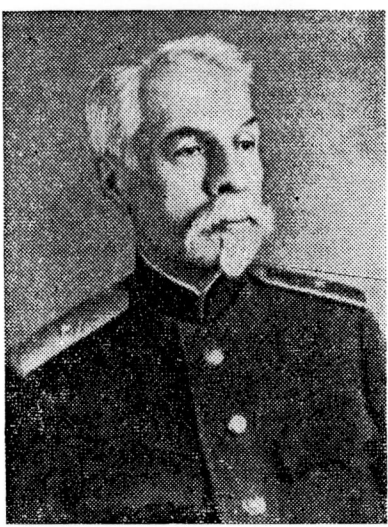

FIGURE 2. Profile of Mikhail Arinkin (Courtesy of Kilinicheskaia Meditsina).

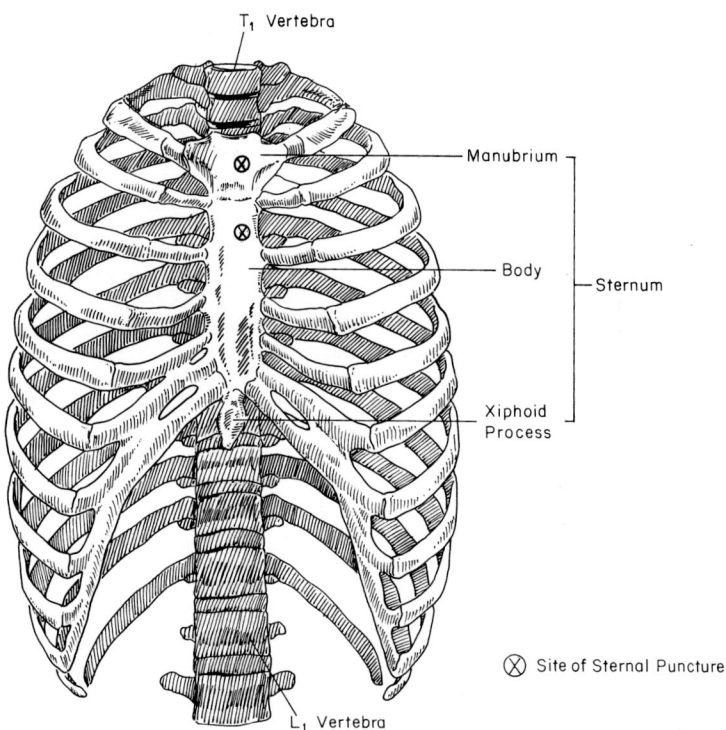

FIGURE 3. Anterior view of the thorax showing anatomical sites of sternal puncture.

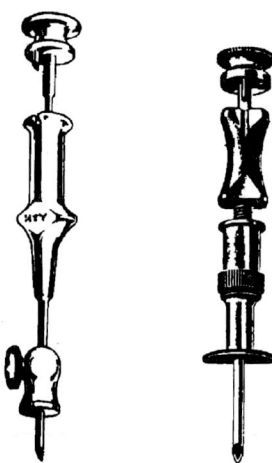

FIGURE 4. Salah (left) and Klima (right) sternal marrow-puncture needle. (Reproduced from Disorders of the Blood by Whitby and Britton (1957), Churchill, London.)

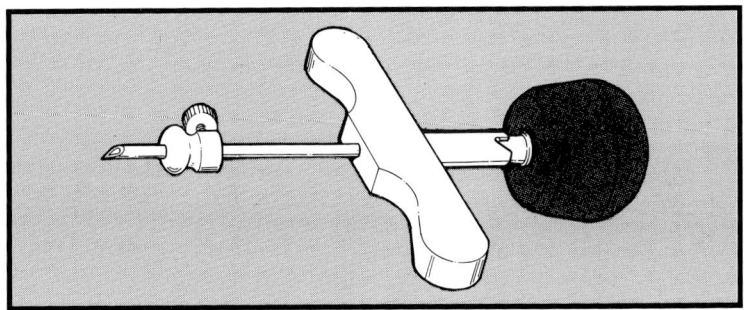

FIGURE 5. The Islam sternal puncture needle.

They were designed in the 1930's and except for the introduction of various kinds of stops and guards there has been very little change over the years in their basic construction and design. These instruments are small, do not conveniently fit the operator's hand, and the lack of a T-bar handle in most instances often makes them difficult to manoeuvre during the sternal puncture procedure. The recently introduced Islam sternal puncture needle (Figure 5) overcomes these disadvantages. The domed handle of its stilette rests comfortably in the operator's hand while the T-bar handle provides a firm grip and precise control of the needle movement. An important feature of the Islam sternal puncture needle is the short length of the penetrating segment (almost one half of a conventional needle, Figure 6).

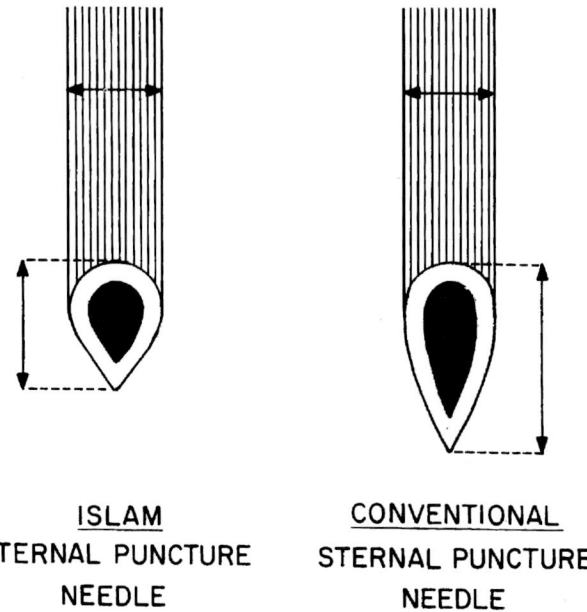

ISLAM
STERNAL PUNCTURE
NEEDLE

CONVENTIONAL
STERNAL PUNCTURE
NEEDLE

FIGURE 6. Penetrating segment of the Islam (left) and conventional (right) sternal puncture needle. (See text for details)

This reduces the possibility of accidental penetration of the inner cortex of the sternum and the subadjacent tissue (pericardium and heart). Further it also has an adjustable guard to prevent accidental excessive penetration and a sloped stop at its expanded proximal end for easy fitting and withdrawal of the stilette.

The Islam Sternal Puncture Needle

The instrument

The instrument* (Figure 7) consists of three parts. The standard size *needle* has an overall length of 45 mm, a uniform external diameter of 2.0 mm and a constant internal diameter of 1.25 mm except for the 2–3 mm distal portion where it is bevelled to produce a tip (cutting edge) very similar to hypodermic needles but much shorter in configuration. The proximal end of the needle has been fitted with a large *metal bar* specifically shaped to insure a firm grip and a standard female luer-lock to receive the nozzle of a syringe and to fit the male luer-lock of the stilette.

---

*The instrument is available in several different sizes (bore diameters) and lengths.

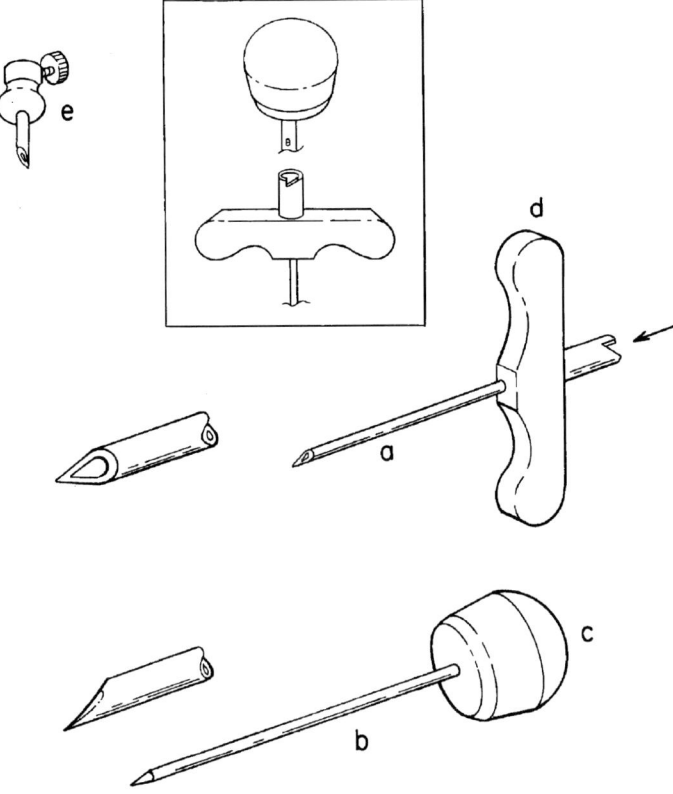

FIGURE 7. Needle (a), stilette (b), dome handle (c), the T-bar handle (d), and the guard (e). The inset shows the details of the luer-lock attachment of the needle and the handle. The sloped stop at the proximal end of the needle is shown by an arrow.

The female luer-lock of the needle also has a sloped stop for easy positioning and resting of the metal stud attached to the male luer-lock of the stilette. This arrangement makes it possible to automatically position the cutting edge of the stilette and needle in the same plane. This design also facilitates the easy unlocking and withdrawal of the stilette (by gentle anti-clockwise rotary motion) during the sternal puncture procedure. As has been mentioned the tip of the needle has been specially designed to make it short (Figure 6) considering the narrowness of the space between the inner and outer plates of the sternum but sharp enough to easily penetrate the overlying soft tissue and bony cortex. The overall length (from the tip to the base, Figure 6) of the penetrating portion of the needle is approximately one half of a conventional needle, thus reducing the fear of accidental penetration of the inner plate of the sternum and injuring the pericardium or heart. The *stilette* is a solid shaft of 1.24 mm in diameter except for the distal portion where it ends in a 2–3 mm bevelled tip to fit the bevelled tip of the needle to provide means of easy penetration of the soft tissue and bony cortex. The proximal end of the stilette has been fitted with a male luer-lock mounted on the inner side of the dome handle to fit the female luer-lock of the needle. It also has a metal stud which fits the sloped stop at the proximal end of the needle and help automatically align the penetrating end of the stilette and needle in the same plane. The proximal end of the stilette is capped with a *smooth dome-shaped solid nylon handle* 25 mm in diameter and 15 mm deep with 5 mm lightly milled edge. It rests snugly in the operator's hand and the two together (the dome and the T-bar handle) provides a uniquely designed instrument to carry out the sternal puncture procedure with efficiency. The metal *guard* is adjustable and can be fixed at any point over the needle by tightening the screw. The adjustable guard is provided mainly to control the depth of penetration during the sternal puncture and also as a precaution and protection against accidents. In obese patients it may be necessary to adjust the guard to a higher level before attempting to enter the sternum. In such circumnstances the positioning of the index finger over the shaft (Figure 8) of the needle helps stabilize the needle and permits adequate control during the sternal puncture procedure. If the sternal puncture needle is used for bone marrow aspiration from sites other than the sternum the adjustable guard may be removed before attempting to penetrate the bone and aspirating the marrow.

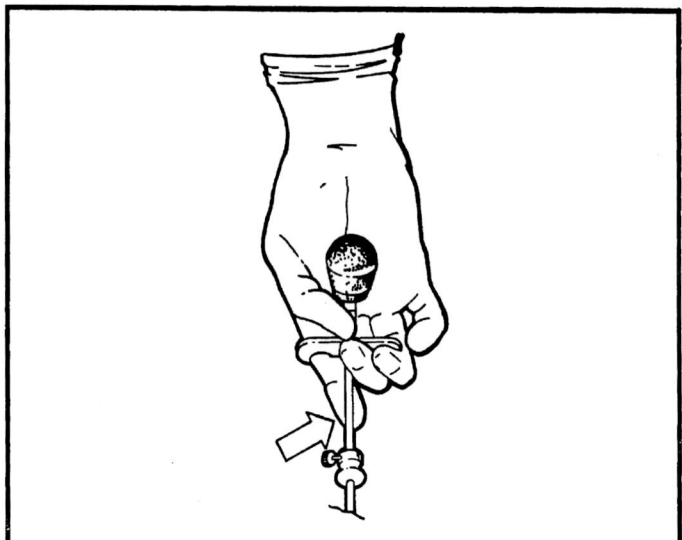

FIGURE 8. Demonstrates the actual holding of the Islam sternal puncture needle. The arrow shows the position of the index finger over the shaft of the needle which helps stabilize the needle and permits adequate control of the needle during the aspiration procedure.

Procedure

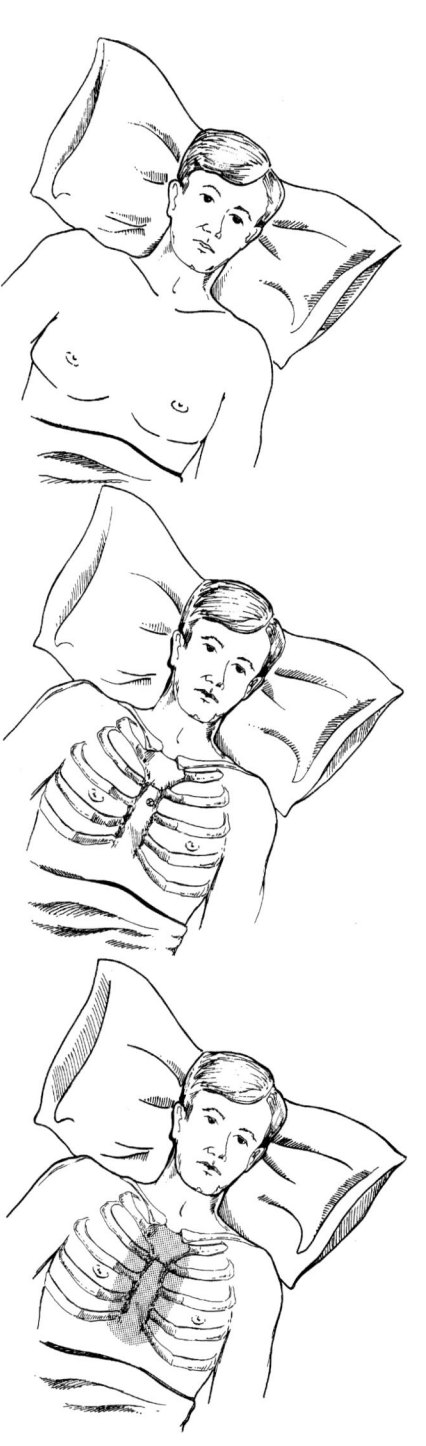

1. Position of the patient: Place the patient on his/her back with the head and neck comfortably resting on a soft low-lying pillow. In men it may be necessary to shave the skin over the sternum prior to puncture.

2. Site: In adult the sternal puncture is usually performed in the proximal region of the body of the sternum, at the level of the second intercostal space, half way between the midsternal line and the left or right sternal border.

3. Identify the area of sternal puncture by palpating the angle of Louis at the junction of the manubrium and body of the sternum. Mark the location with an indelible marker or digital pressure. Surgically prepare the area down to the fourth intercostal space with alcohol and iodine and then drape the site.

4. First withdraw 3–5 ml of anaesthetic (2% lignocane) through a 21 gauge 1 1/2″ needle into a 5 ml syringe. Then substitute the 21 gauge needle for a 25 gauge 5/8″ hypodermic needle and make an intradermal injection producing a 5 mm papule. Replace the 25 gauge with a 21 gauge needle and pass it through the papule infiltrating the subcutaneous tissue with the local anaesthetic. Then with the needle still in place also inject about 1.0 ml directly into the periosteum. Give ample time for the anaesthetic to take effect.

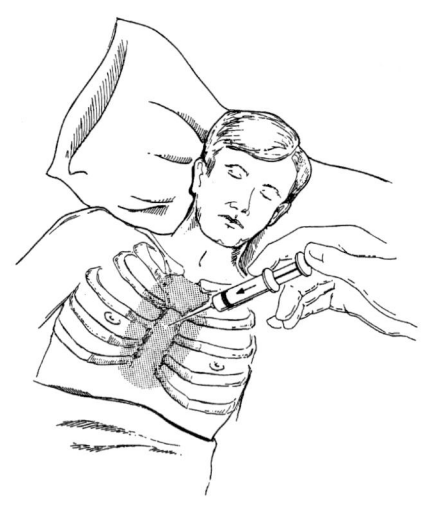

5. It is useful to probe the site with a 21 gauge, one and a half inch needle (with or without an attached syringe) to roughly assess the effect of the anaesthetiche and the depth at which the sternum will be struck. Using this as a guide, adjust and firmly fix the guard on to the shaft of the bone marrow aspiration needle.

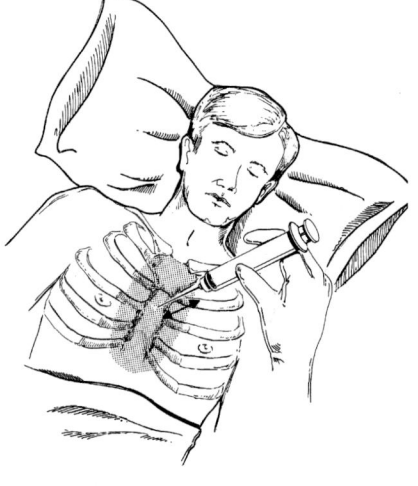

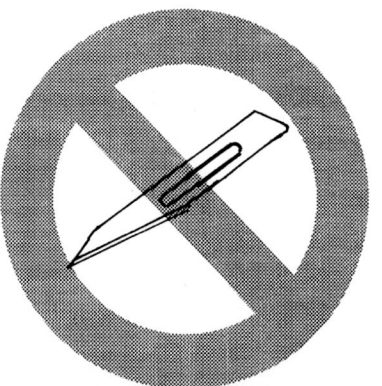

6. No skin incision is necessary for this procedure.

7. Hold the needle assembly with the domed handle in the palm, the middle and fourth fingers over the transverse handle, and the index finger against the shaft of the needle. The position of the index finger against the shaft (arrow) helps stabilize the needle and controls it during the sternal puncture procedure.

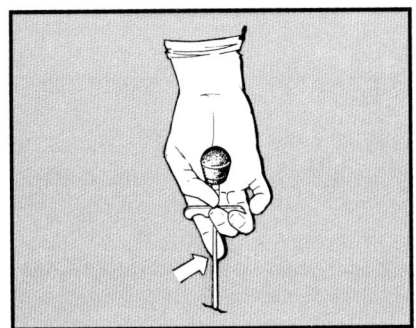

8. After skin sterilisation and local anaesthesia of the skin, subcutaneous tissue and periosteum the needle with its stilette in place is slowly and gently advanced towards the sternum so as to hit the bone at a right angle (or at 45°). When the sternum is reached it is then penetrated by gentle rotary (clockwise/counterclockwise) motion of the needle.

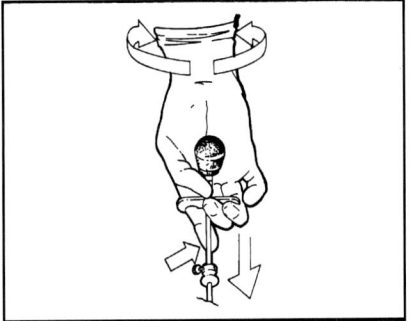

9. Entrance into the sternal marrow cavity is recognised by a "sudden" give of the needle which indicates that the outer table of the sternum has been perforated. Once the cortex is penetrated advance the needle only few milimeters into the marrow cavity with gentle, reciprocal clockwise/counterclockwise rotary motion.

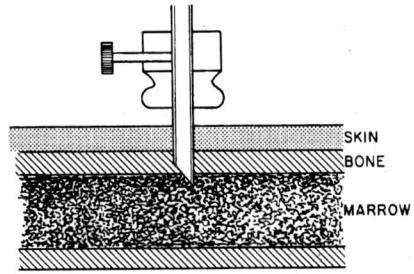

10. Once the needle is in place — hold it in position with the left hand, (as shown in the illustration), unlock the stilette and domed handle by anticlockwise twist and gently remove it.

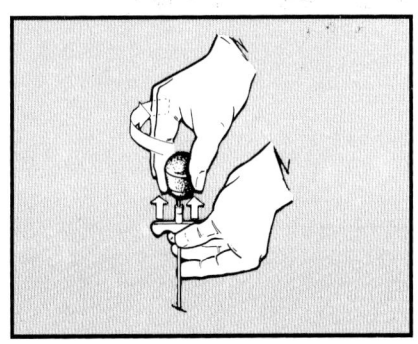

11. Attach a syringe to the needle mount.

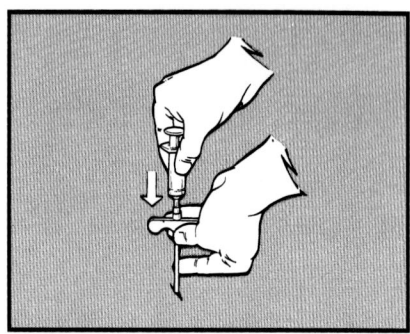

12. Apply a negative pressure and aspirate the required amount of marrow sample from the sternum.

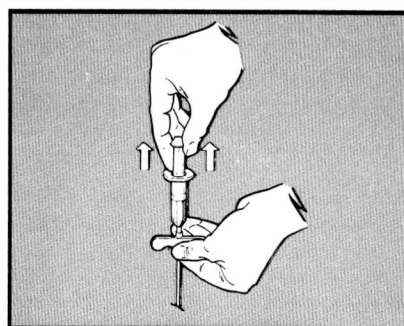

13. Following aspiration of the required amount marrow remove the syringe from the needle mount and using sterile technique, close the proximal opening of the needle (arrow) to prevent any loss of marrow or blood from the wound while the marrow specimen collected in the syringe is being delivered into a bottle containing EDTA (or other anticoagulant) for processing and examination.

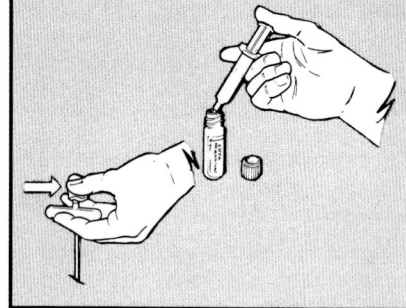

14. Replace and lock the stilette with domed handle by a twisting clockwise motion.

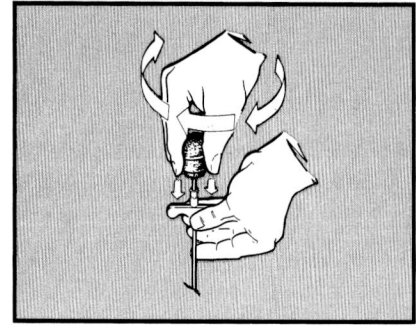

15. Slowly withdraw the needle with the right hand with a gentle alternating rotary motion while fixing the sternum with the index and middle fingers of the left hand.

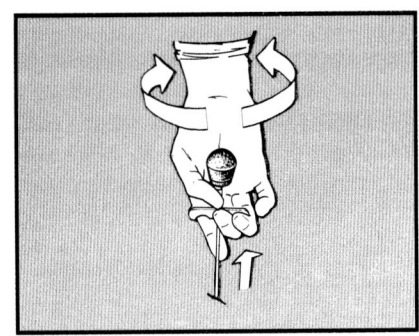

16. After withdrawal of the needle, apply firm pressure for one or two minutes over the site of the puncture to prevent any bleeding and then cover the wound with a small dressing.

Note: To protect the marrow aspiration needle and obtain the desired results the needle should never be introduced or withdrawn without the stilette in place.

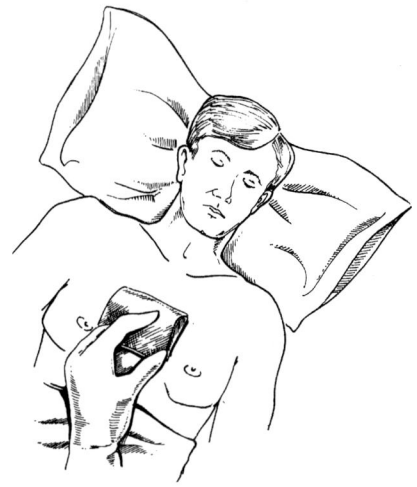

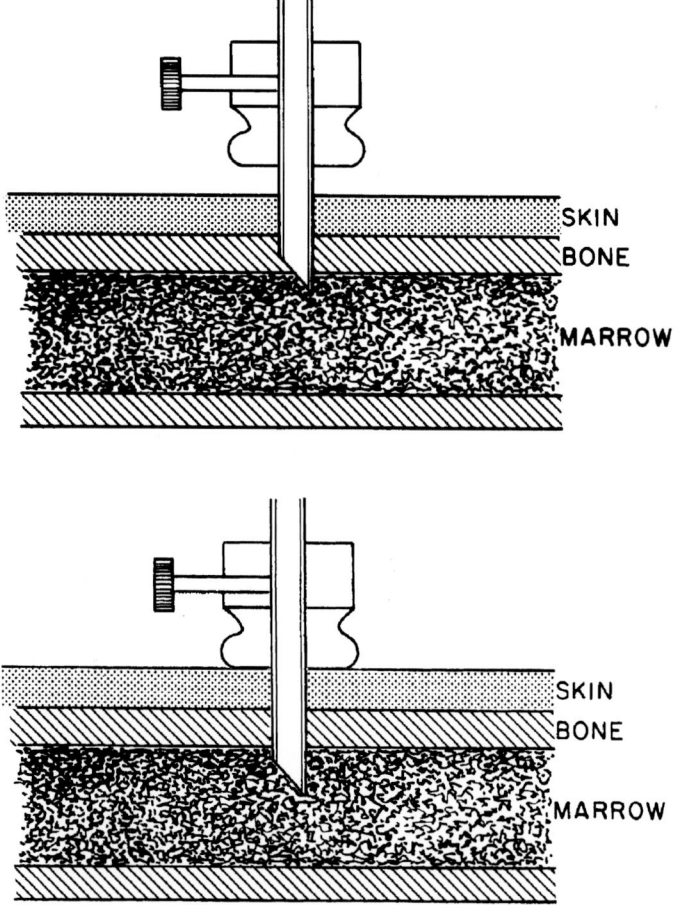

FIGURE 9. Schematic representation of the sternal puncture procedure using the Islam sternal puncture needle.

Schematic Representation of the Sternal Puncture Procedure Using the Islam Sternal Puncture Needle

1. The sternal puncture needle, with the stilette and handle in place and the guard firmly secured at a proper distance from the distal end of the needle, is slowly advanced through the skin and subcutaneous tissue towards the sternum so as to hit the bone at 90°. When the sternum is reached, it is gently penetrated by clockwise and counterclockwise rotary motion of the needle (Figure 9, upper).
2. Once the outer table of the sternum is penetrated the needle is advanced slowly a few milimeters in the marrow cavity by the same rotary motion of the needle (Figure 9, lower).

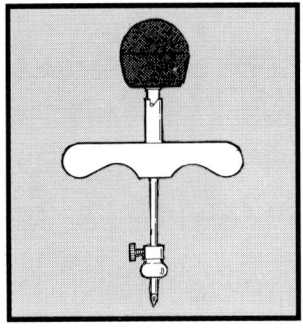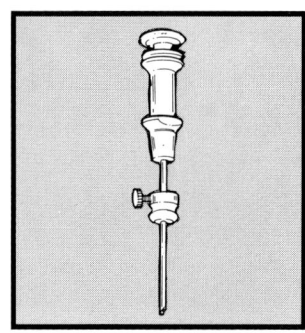

FIGURE 10. Islam (left) and conventional (right) sternal puncture needle.

3. Once the needle is in place within the marrow cavity, the stilette is removed with an anti-clockwise twisting action, a syringe is attached, and the aspiration performed.
4. Following aspiration of the desired amount of bone marrow, the stilette is promptly replaced and adequately secured and the whole needle assembly is withdrawn with a rotary motion.

Difference Between Conventional and Islam Sternal Puncture Needle

Conventional sternal puncture needles (Figure 10, right) are small, do not fit properly in the operators hand, and due to the absence in most instances, of a T-bar handle, are often difficult to manoeuvre during the sternal puncture procedure.

The recently introduced Islam sternal puncture needles (Figure 10, left) are larger, stronger and more effective in obtaining bone marrow aspirate samples from the sternum than the conventional sternal puncture needles. The large T-bar handle permits a secure and firm grip and the smooth dome shaped handle rests snugly in the operators hand providing a comfortable cushion during the sternal puncture procedure. These two important features (the T-bar and the dome handle) are lacking in the conventional sternal puncture needles. In addition, in the Islam sternal puncture needle the penetrating end of the needle has been designed to make it sharp and relatively broad but not overtly long to insure the penetration of the outer but not the inner lamina of the sternum while retaining the aspirating end of the needle within the narrow medullary space of the sternum.

Precaution

Although the technique of sternal puncture is a safe and very effective method of diagnostic marrow aspiration, care must be taken while performing this procedure on elderly patients, particularly elderly women who may have severe osteoporosis.

Bone manifesting this pathology lacks normal density and may permit a diagnostic needle to penetrate deeper than desired even with normal pressure. The sternum should never be punctured below the second intercostal space, because, at the level of the third and fourth intercostal spaces, the sternum lies in close proximity to the pericardium and heart.

During sternal puncture procedure the patient may become apprehensive as the needle is being introduced into the chest. It is advisable to inform the patient fully about the entire procedure (including the momentary and fleeting suction pain) before it is undertaken in order to reduce the fear and anxiety. It is also advisable to practice on cadavers to obtain confidence and experience in this procedure.

ILIAC PUNCTURE

The ilium (Figure 11) is another site from which haematopoietic marrow may be withdrawn. The ilium can be penetrated without much difficulty in a variety of places; the crest, however, offers too great resistance for it to be a practical site for routine penetration except perhaps in infants and children in whom the compact bone is less hard. Usually the site near the anterior superior iliac spine (anterior iliac puncture) or the area near the posterior superior iliac spine (posterior iliac puncture) is chosen for aspirating bone marrow samples from this bone. It should be noted that the ilium offers greater resistance to penetration than the sternum and consequently stronger needles are required for this approach.

Anterior Iliac Puncture (Figure 12)

For puncture of the anterior iliac crest, the area just posterior to the anterior superior iliac spine is utilised. Some haematologists prefer the area about 1–2 cm inferior to the crest and 1–2 cm posterior to the anterior superior iliac spine. Others have found more success with an area about 1 cm below the crest and about 1 or 2 cm posterior to the anterior gluteal line. At the anterior iliac crest the compact bone frequently proves to be exceedingly hard, so that the entire aspiration needle sometimes bends and is also inclined to slip off the site.

Instrumentation

Both the Salah and Klima needles as well as the Islam sternal puncture needle can be used for obtaining bone marrow aspirate samples from the anterior iliac crest. The Salah and Klima needles however, were originally designed for the sternum, a much softer bone. They are potentially weaker and less suitable for puncture of the harder ilium where the needle may be at risk. The Islam sternal puncture needles

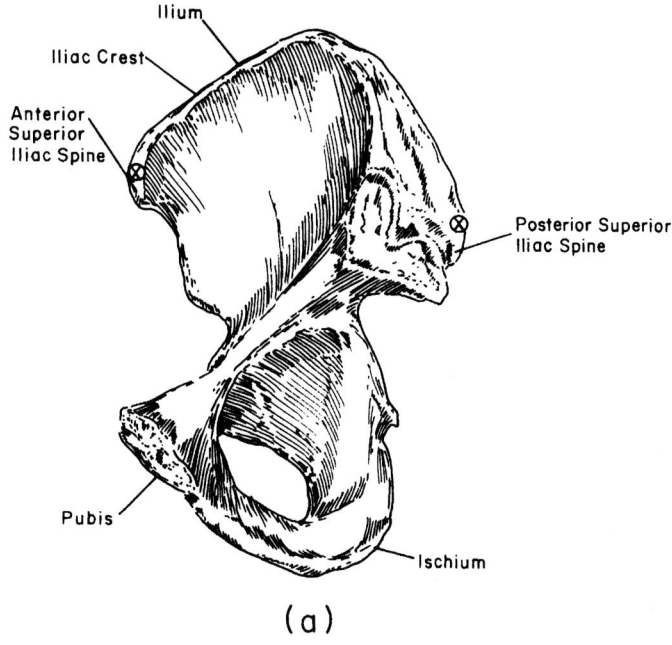

(a)

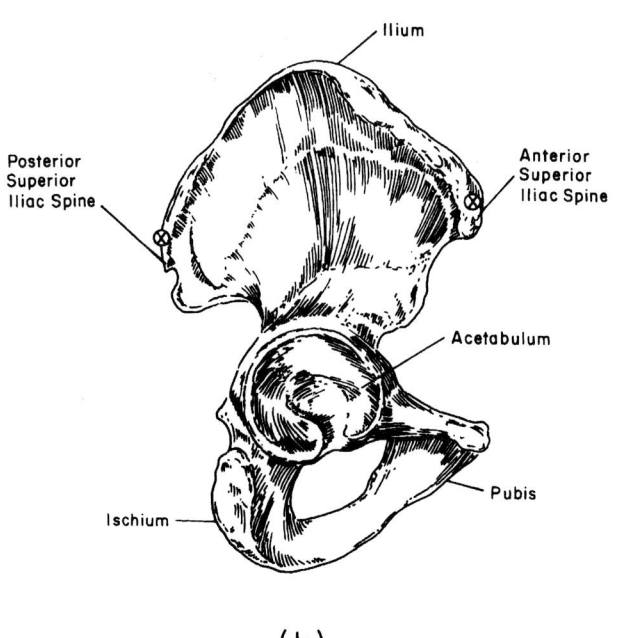

(b)

FIGURE 11. Illustrations of the ilium: (a) internal surface, (b) external surface, and the usual sites of bone marrow aspiration. ⊗ = site of aspiration.

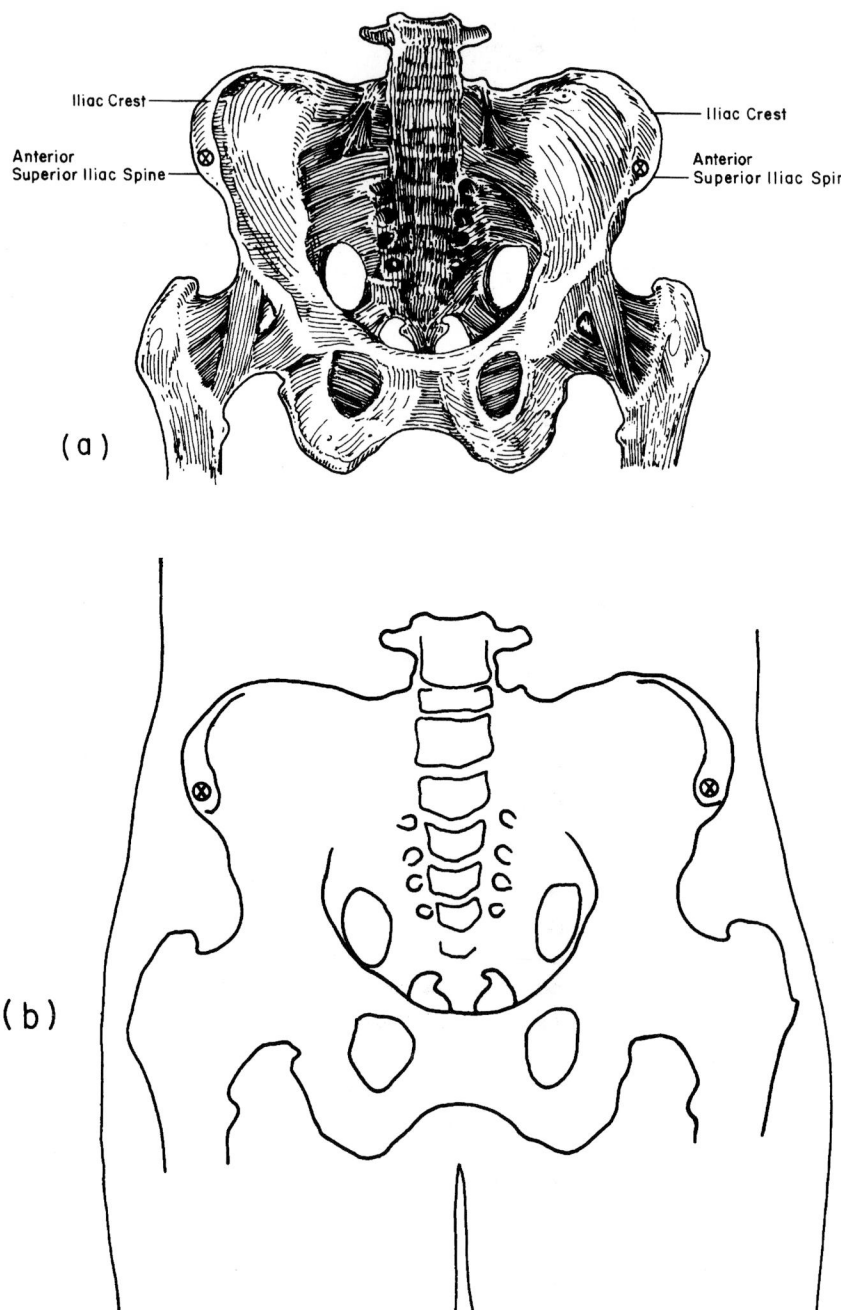

FIGURE 12. (a) Anterior view of the pelvis, (b) pelvis *in situ*. ⊗ = site of anterior iliac puncture.

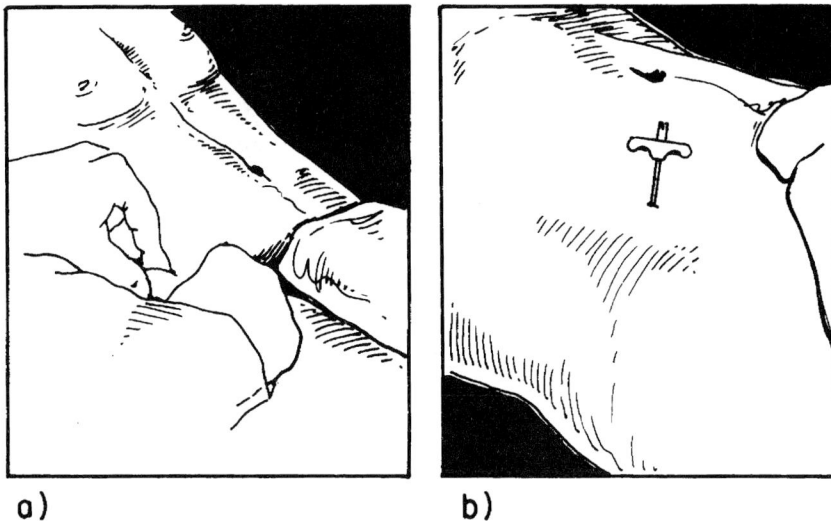

a)   b)

FIGURE 13. (a) The oval protuberance near the anterior superior iliac spine is located between the thumb and forefinger. (b) The needle is introduced perpendicularly (or pointing slightly cephalically) into the ilium.

are much sturdier and due to the presence of a T-bar and dome handle it is easier to hold and manoeuvre during puncture of a hard bone. Depending on the operator's preferences the Islam needle may well be the needle best suited for anterior iliac puncture.

Procedure

The patient should lie flat on a reasonably firm surface. The site typically punctured is just behind the anterior superior iliac spine. It is located with the fingers as an oval protuberance (Figure 13a). Using sterile technique the skin is prepared with an antiseptic and draped. The skin, subcutaneous tissue and periosteum are infiltrated with a local anaesthetic. Ample time should be given for the anaesthetic to take effect. It is useful to probe the site with a 21 gauge, $1\frac{1}{2}$ inch needle to roughly outline the borders of anterior iliac crest and to ascertain the effect of the anaesthetic. This also gives an indication of the depth at which the bone will be struck and also permits determination of the proper angulation of the needle. With the patient in the supine position as indicated, and the anterior iliac crest properly secured by the thumb and forefingers of the left hand, the needle is introduced perpendicularly (or pointing slightly cephalically) into the ilium (Figure 13b). If the Islam sternal puncture needle is used, the guard should be removed and the needle assembly held with the domed handle in the palm, the middle and fourth fingers over the

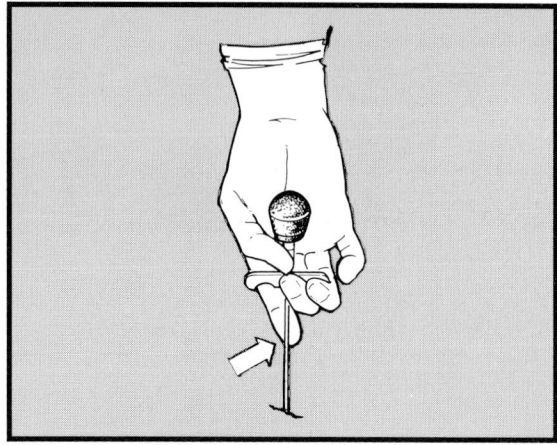

FIGURE 14. Demonstration of the holding of the Islam sternal puncture needle during anterior iliac puncture.

transverse handle, and the index finger over the shaft of the needle (Figure 14). The position of the index finger over the shaft (arrow) helps stabilize the needle and facilitates positive control of its movements.

Posterior Iliac Puncture (Figure 15)

The area of the posterior iliac spine is the thickest region of the ilium and houses the largest volume of haematopoietic (red) marrow both in the child and in the adult. It is easily acccessible and large amounts of red marrow are readily aspirated. This segment of the ilium is distant from any vital structure and hence complications are unlikely. The patient also cannot observe the procedure and the anxiety often associated with a sternal puncture is thus avoided. An additional favourable feature is the fact that the cortical bone at this region is also appreciably less dense than it is in the area of the anterior iliac spine and thus more easily penetrable.

Instrumentation

The Salah and Klima needles have been commonly used for posterior (as well as anterior) iliac bone marrow aspiration. As indicated, they were initially designed to obtain sternal samples of marrow and are not particularly suited for iliac puncture where the configuration of the bone is different and the thickness of the cortex is greater.

The Islam posterior iliac puncture needles (Figure 16) have been specifically designed to obtain bone marrow aspirate samples from the posterior iliac crests.

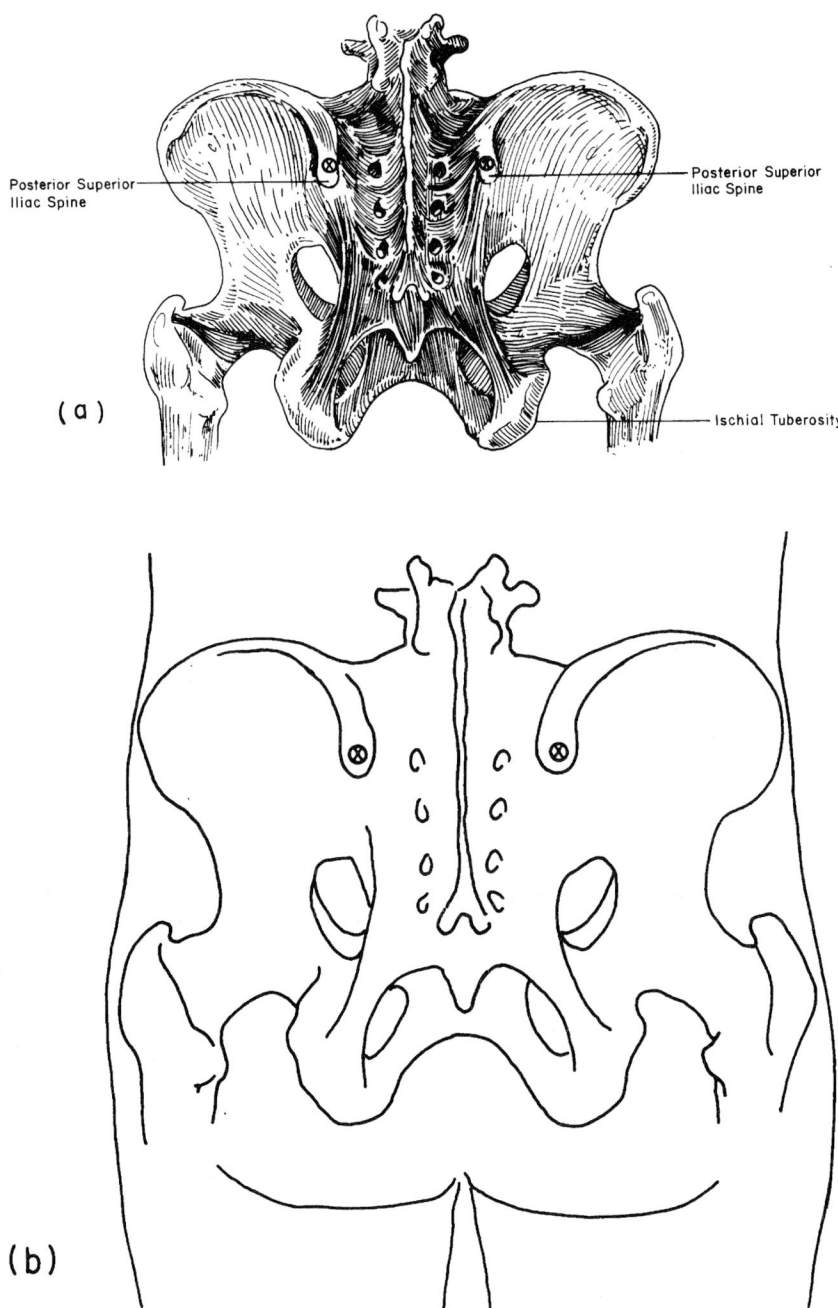

Posterior Superior Iliac Spine

Posterior Superior Iliac Spine

Ischial Tuberosity

(a)

(b)

FIGURE 15. (a) Pelvis, posterior view (b) pelvis *in situ*. ⊗ = Site of posterior iliac puncture.

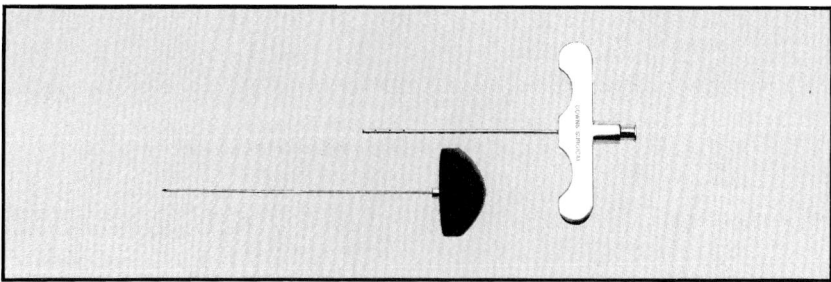

FIGURE 16. The Islam posterior iliac puncture needle. (This needle is also available with side holes near the frontal opening).

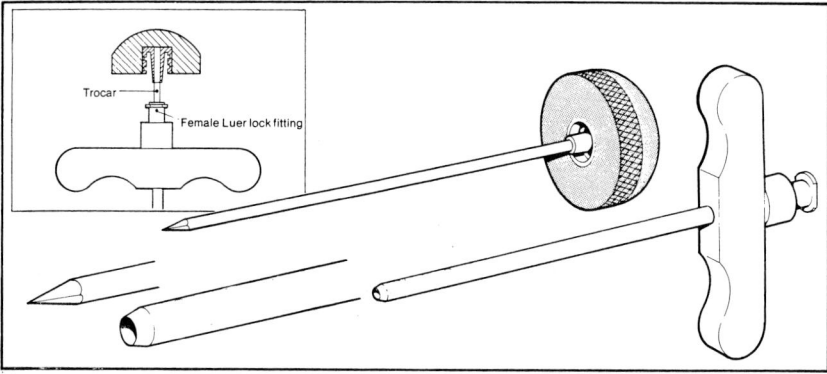

FIGURE 17. Illustration of the details of the Islam posterior iliac puncture needle without side holes. The needle (a), stilette (b) and the dome handle (c). The inset shows the details of the luer lock attachment of the needle and the handle.

These instruments are longer and stronger than the conventional aspiration needles, and the presence of a T-bar and domed handle makes them much easier to hold and manoeuvre during the aspiration procedure.

The Standard size steel instrument* (Figure 17) consists of two parts. (a) *The needle* has an overall length of 80 mm , a uniform external diameter of 2.35 mm and a constant internal diameter of 1.78 mm except for the 1.25 mm distal portion where it is bevelled to 18°. The proximal end of the needle has been fitted with a large metal bar specially shaped for firm grip and a female luer lock to receive the nozzle of a syringe and to fit the male luer lock of the stilette and domed handle. (b) *The stilette* is a solid shaft 1.62 mm in diameter except for the distal portion where it ends with a 3.0 mm long, three faceted, sharp-pointed cutting

---

*Other sizes (bore diameters) and lengths are also available.

tip which projects beyond the distal end of the needle to provide a means of easy penetration of the soft tissue and bony cortex. The proximal end of the stilette has been mounted into a male luer lock buried inside the dome handle to fit the female luer lock of the needle. The proximal end of the stilette has been capped with a hemispherical smooth dome-shaped solid nylon handle (c) 30 mm in diameter and 15 mm deep with a 5 mm lightly milled edge. It has been designed to rest snugly in the operator's hand and to provide comfort if and when forceful thrusting is necessary.

Aspiration Procedure

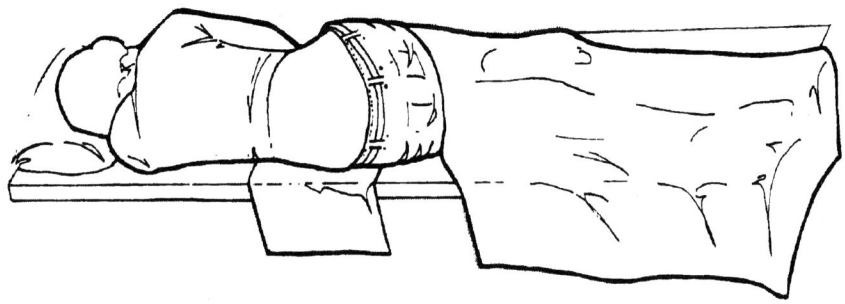

1. Position of the patient — The patient is placed in a right or left lateral decubitus position, with the knees drawn up and back comfortably flexed, or in the prone position with pillow beneath the hips.

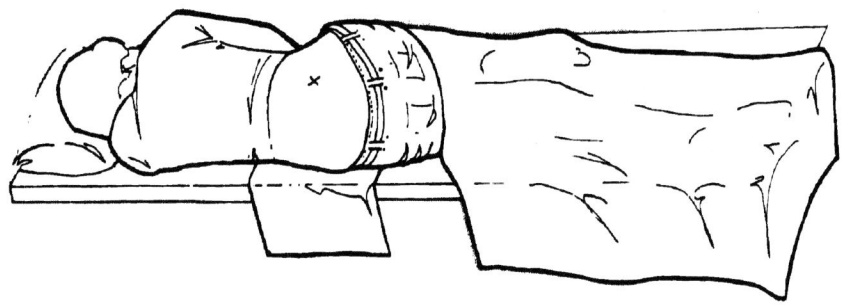

2. Locate the posterior iliac crest by palpation and mark the area with indelible marker or thumbnail pressure. With the use of sterile technique prepare the skin with an antiseptic and drape.

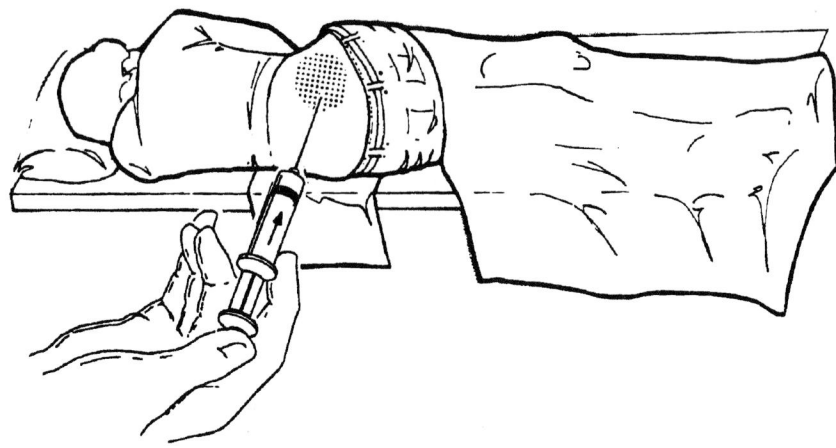

3. First infiltrate the skin with the anaesthetic using a small 25 gauge 5/8″ hypodermic needle. After few seconds infiltrate the subcutaneous tissue, muscle and periosteum with the same local anaesthetic entering the tissue through the same puncture wound but using a larger 21 gauge $1\frac{1}{2}''$ hypodermic needle. Provide ample time for the anaesthetic to take effect.

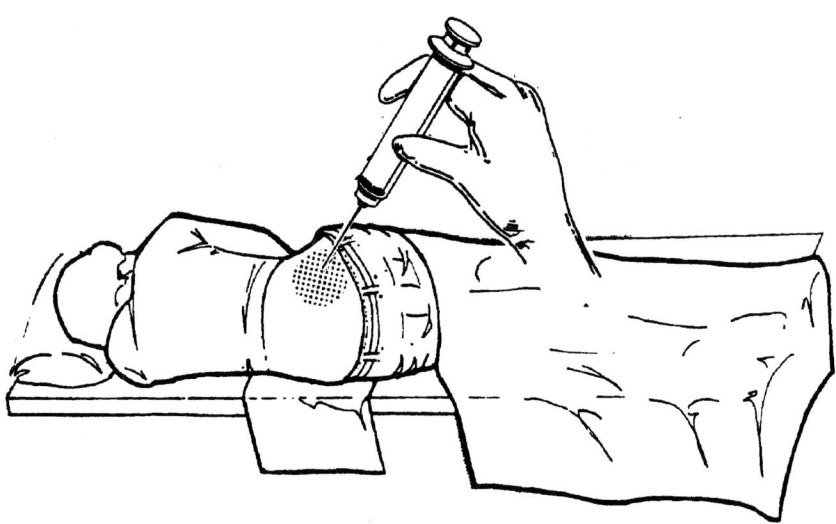

4. It is always useful to probe the aspiration site with a 21 gauge $1\frac{1}{2}''$ needle to establish whether the anaesthetic has taken affect and to roughly outline the borders of posterior iliac crest. This technique also gives an indication as to the depth at which the bone will be struck and also permits determination of the proper angulation of the needle.

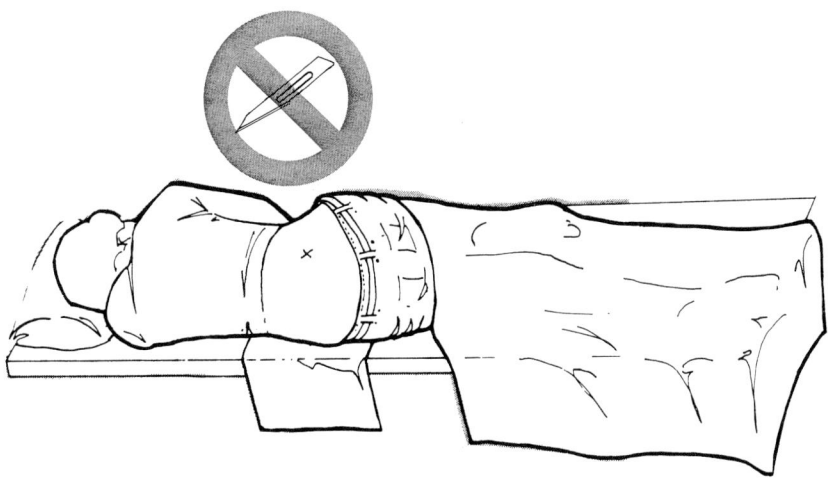

5. No skin incision is usually necessary for this procedure. However, if a solid tissue bone marrow biopsy is also to be performed at the same site following aspiration of the marrow, a skin incision would be preferable.

6. Holding of the needle — Hold the needle assembly with the domed handle in the palm, middle and fourth fingers over the transverse handle, and the index finger against the shaft of the needle. The position of the index finger over the shaft (arrow) helps stabilize the needle and permits adequate control during penetration of the soft and bony tissues.

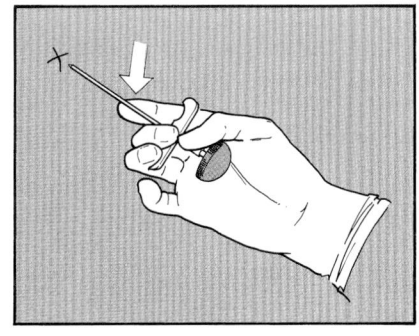

7. With the stilette and domed handle in place — introduce the needle through the skin and slowly advance it towards the surface of the posterior ilium pointing the needle in the direction of the anterior superior iliac spine. When the posterior iliac crest is reached, penetrate the cortical bone with gentle rotary motions of the needle.

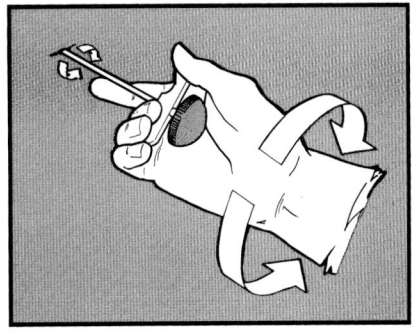

8. Once the cortex is penetrated (which can be felt by decreased resistance) — slowly advance the needle into the marrow cavity with gentle clockwise-anticlockwise rotary motions until an adequate depth (0.5–1.0 cm) is reached.

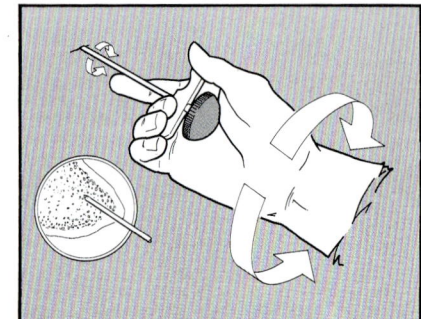

9. Once the needle is in place — hold it in position with the left hand (as shown in the illustration), unlock the stilette and domed handle by anti-clockwise twist and gently remove it.

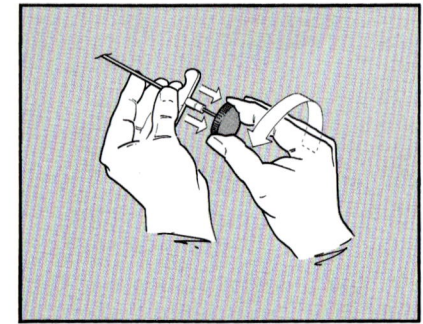

10. Attach a syringe on to the needle mount. Apply a negative pressure and aspirate the required amount of marrow sample.

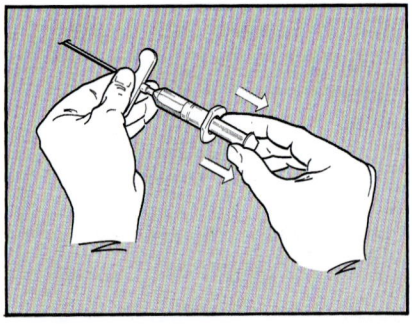

11. Following aspiration of the marrow remove the syringe from the needle. Using sterile technique close the proximal opening of the needle (arrow) to prevent any exudation of marrow from the patient while the collected sample in the syringe is delivered into a container with anti-coagulant (e.g. EDTA) or other receptacle(s) for processing and examination. It is during these maneuvers that an assistant is particularly helpful.

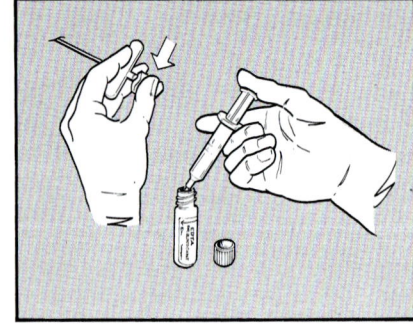

12. Once the aspiration is complete replace the stilette with domed handle and lock it with the neelde by twisting clockwise.

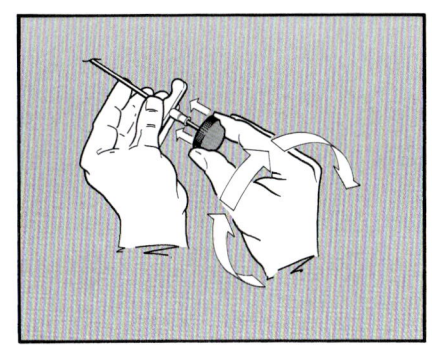

13. Then slowly withdraw the needle by gentle alternating rotary motions. Firmly hold the shaft, T-bar and domed handle together during the withdrawal.

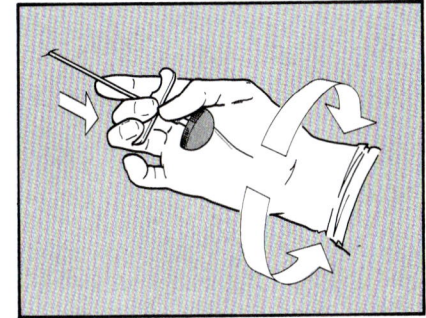

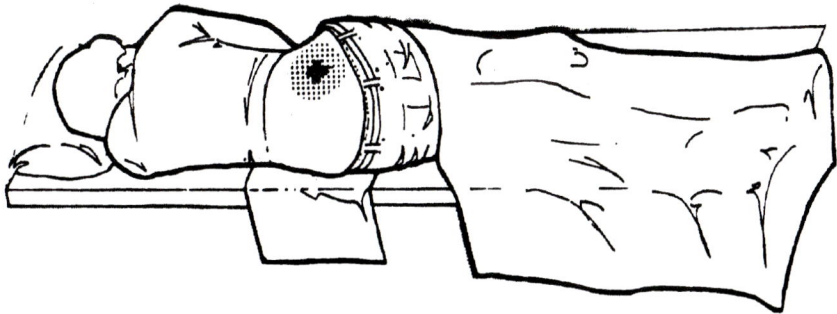

14. After withdrawal of the needle apply firm pressure for one or two minutes at the puncture site to prevent any bleeding and then cover the wound with a small sterile dressing.

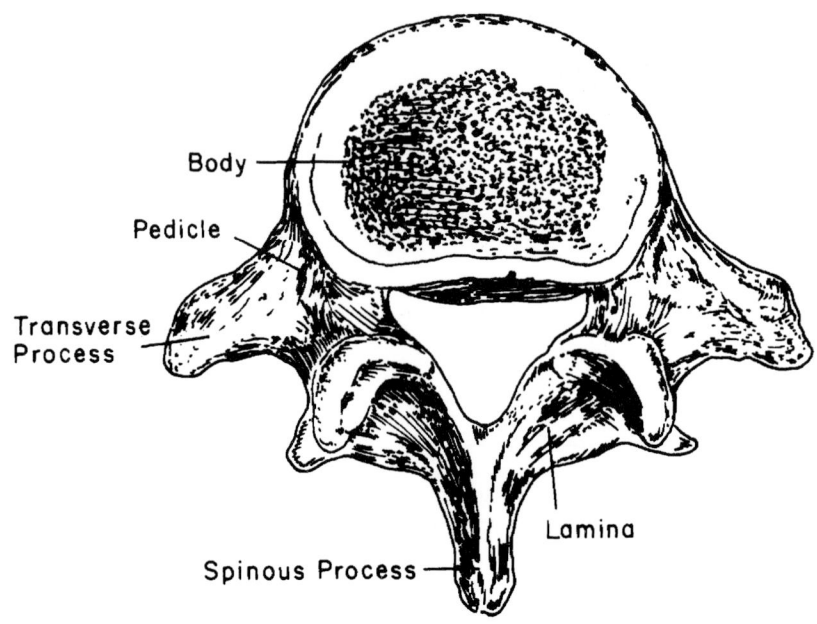

FIGURE 18. A lumbar vertebra showing its spinous process.

PUNCTURE OF SPINOUS PROCESSES OF LUMBAR VERTEBRAE (FIGURE 18)

Adequate samples of marrow may be obtained from adults by puncturing the spinous processes of lumbar vertebrae. Although punctures are not too difficult at the spinous process(es) because of their superficial location and ease of identification, the volume of marrow available for aspiration is limited. The sternum and posterior ilium, thus remain the most generous sites for obtaining samples of haematopoietic (red) marrow.

Instrumentation

Any of the available sternal puncture needles can be used for puncturing the spinous processes of lumbar vertebrae. Conventional needles however are rather small and thus can be inconvenient to hold and manoeuvre with precision. The Islam sternal puncture needles are an optimal choice for this approach. The T-bar and domed handle facilate a comfortable grip and positive, accurate penetration of the bone. They are also available in several different sizes (bore diameters) and lengths. Thus depending on the physical size of the patient an appropriate size and length of the needle may be selected.

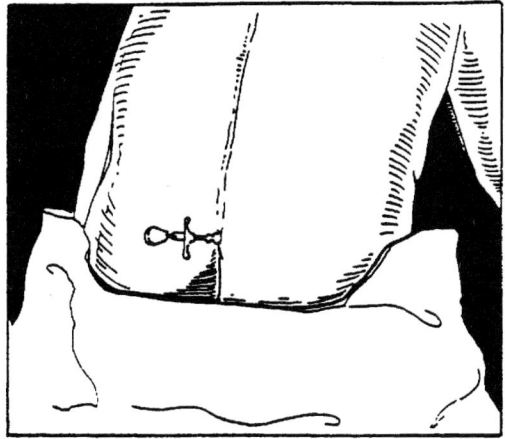

FIGURE 19. Demonstrates lumbar spinal process puncture. The patient is in a sitting position with the back comfortably flexed. An Islam sternal puncture needle is fixed in the spinous process of a lumbar vertebra.

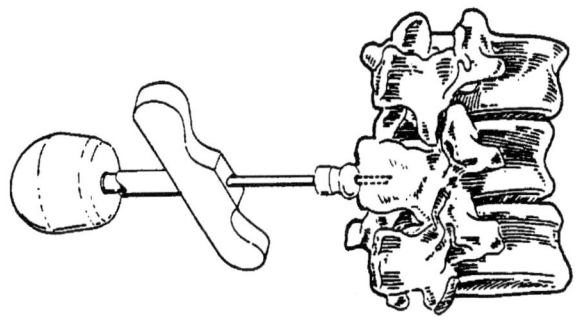

FIGURE 20. Lumbar vertebrae 2,3 and 4 with an Islam sternal puncture needle fixed in the spinous process of L3.

Procedure

The patient is placed in a right or left lateral decubitus position with the knees drawn up and back comfortably flexed or in a sitting position as for a lumbar puncture (Figures 19, 20). The lumbar spinous process to be punctured is located and marked with an indelible pen or thumb nail pressure. Following the usually accepted precautions of skin sterilization and local anaesthesia, the needle with its stilette in place is slowly advanced through the skin and subcutaneous tissue in the mid-line and at right angles to the skin surface pointing towards the spinous process. Once the spinous process is reached the needle is introduced into the spine

Puncture to the Tibia

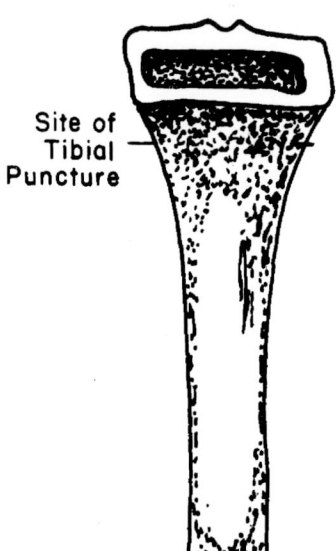

Site of
Tibial —
Puncture

FIGURE 21. Diagram of the tibia in later childhood, indicating the optimal site for tibial (marrow) puncture.

with gentle rotary motions. When the needle is in place the stilette is removed, a syringe is attached, and the aspiration is performed. Following aspiration, the stilette is promptly replaced and the needle is withdrawn firmly holding the shaft and T-bar together. After withdrawal of the needle local pressure is applied to prevent any bleeding and then a small sterile dressing is applied.

PUNCTURE OF THE TIBIA (FIGURE 21)

The tibia contains active marrow at its proximal (epiphyseal) end throughout the entire childhood. Haematopoietic marrow has been successfully aspirated from the tibia in children at the age of 10 years. It is the accepted practice to select the tibia as the preferred site of puncture in all children under the age of 2 years.

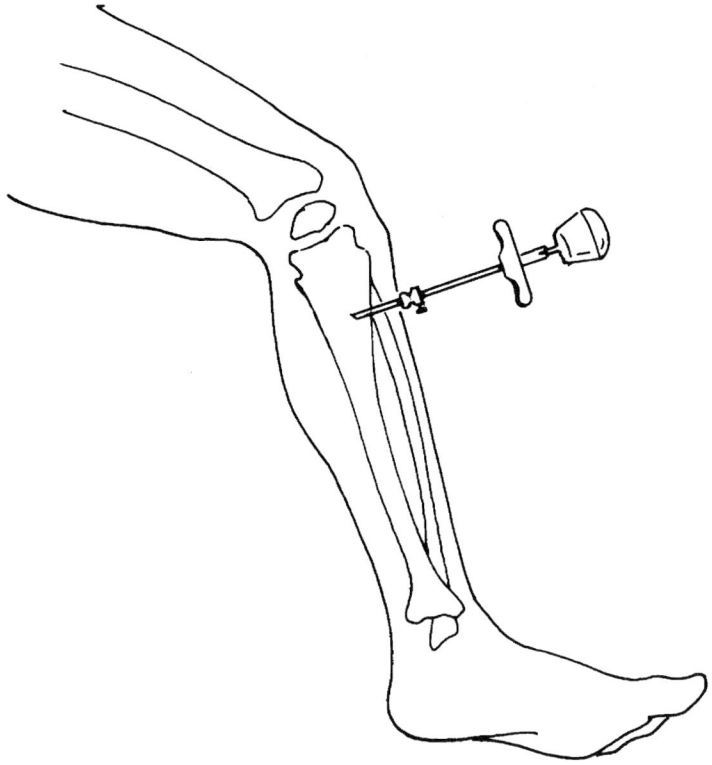

FIGURE 22. Schematic demonstration of a tibial puncture procedure.

Instrumentation

Any of the available sternal puncture needles can be used for puncturing the tibia. Salah, Klima or similar needles may be used. The Islam sternal puncture needles are ideally suited for this purpose because of their improved design and ease of manipulation.

Aspiration Procedure

The flat triangular, non-muscular area on the medial aspect of the proximal end of the tibia is the site usually selected for aspiration of haematopoietic bone marrow from this long bone (Figure 22). The best point for the insertion of needle appears to be medial to the insertion of the patellar tendon at the tibial tuberosity. This site is often the only certain, dependable landmark in an obese infant. If the needle is inserted lower in the shaft, difficulty is likely to be experienced due to thickening of the bony cortex and narrowing of the lumen of the medullary cavity.

ASPIRATION FROM OTHER SITES

As previously mentioned, almost any area of functioning marrow near the surface of the body may be utilised for obtaining a bone marrow aspirate. The two most commonly used sites are the sternum (at the level of the second intercostal space), and the posterior iliac crest. However, other bones such as ribs, vertebral bodies, tibia and femer (or other bones if accessible by an aspirating needle) may be used particularly when there is radiologic evidence of a bone lesion. In such circumstances aspiration of marrow from a lesion may be aided by prior localisation of the site ("hot spots") with radionuclide or other imaging techniques. This is particularly true in certain haematologic and non-haematologic malignant conditions (e.g. multiple myeloma and metastatic breast carcinoma respectively).

CHOICE OF PUNCTURE SITE(S)

In general, the overall composition (cellularity, myeloid-erythroid ratio, cytomorphology) of marrow withdrawn from a bone containing haematopoietic marrow is usually similar regardless of the bone selected for study. Which site is used is a matter of personal preference. It should be noted, however, there can be considerable variation even in adjacent sites particularly under pathologic conditions. Such cellular manifestations are more likely to be recognised when aspiration biopsies are accompanied by concomitant histologic sections.

The sternum is probably the easiest bone to puncture and does indeed yield very satisfactory samples. As a result the sternum remains one of the most commonly utilised aspiration sites. It does nevertheless have disadvantages. First, the patient is aware of the activities surrounding him or her and can observe the entire procedure. Apprehension, especially when the needle is introduced into the sternum is to be expected. Second, deaths have been reported due to cardiovascular penetration (such risks are extremely small in adults when the procedure is performed carefully and with a guard firmly in place on the shaft of the needle). With these precautions the incidence of serious risk should be reduced to zero. Third, the sternum contains a relatively small volume of marrow which, though usually sufficient for most diagnostic requirements, may not be adequate when large amounts of aspirate are desired.

The advent of improved needles designed for the aspiration of marrow from the posterior ilium has permitted this site to be ideal and perhaps even preferable to sternum. It is readily accessible, large amounts of marrow can be obtained, and is distant from any vital structures. Complications are unlikely and as the patient cannot observe the procedure, anxiety is avoided.

THE MULTIPORT ASPIRATION NEEDLE

The technique of examination of bone narrow aspirates obtained via conventional marrow aspiration needles is widely used in the diagnosis of malignant and benign,

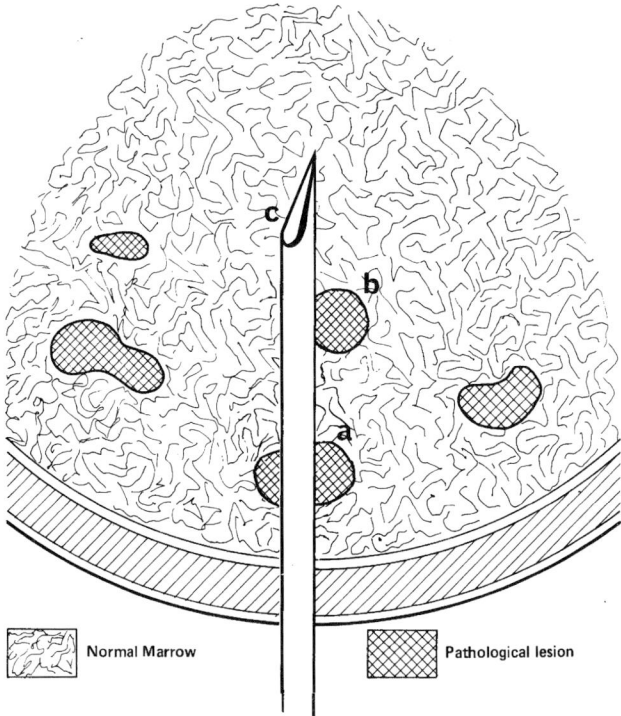

FIGURE 23. Schematic representation of the aspiration procedure by a conventional aspiration needle. It shows that the needle with the stilette in place, has gone through a lesion during insertion (a), by-passed a lesion (b) and lodged its frontal opening into an area of normal marrow (c).

haematologic and non-haematologic conditions. Inherent in the structure of such needles, though almost totally unappreciated, is the fact that marrow fragments are only obtained from a limited volume of tissue near the open front end (mouth) of the needle.

Bone marrow has patchy, random involvment in many pathological processes, a feature documented by multiple marrow aspiration studies in selected patients. Conventional aspiration needles have only one opening for the access and sampling of marrow. Their sampling may or may not include cells near to or distant from the point of aspiration (Figure 23). To help eliminate the uncertainty of obtaining cells from distant and separate loci of pathology a multi pore aspiration needle has been designed. The use of this instrument reduces the risk of failure to sample small focal infiltrates in conditions as lymphoma, leukaemia, preleukaemia (MDS), and metastatic malignancy (Figure 24). Experience has further indicated this needle is particularly useful in posterior ilial (posterior iliac crest) aspirations because of the enhanced depth of penetration afforded by this bone.

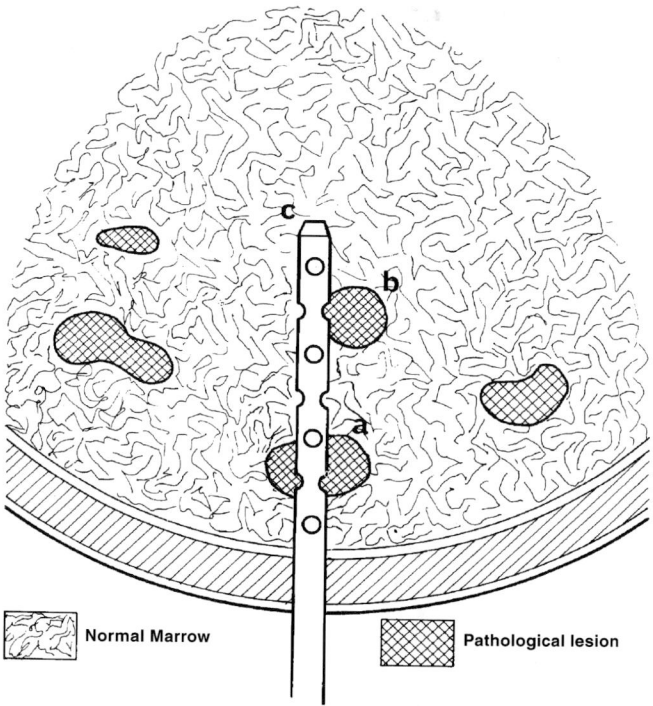

FIGURE 24. Schematic representation of the aspiration procedure performed with a multiple port bone marrow aspiration needle. It shows that the needle with the stilette in place has gone through a lesion during insertion (a), by-passed another lesion (b) in the same manner as the conventional needle in Figure 23 with the terminal opening lodged in an area of normal marrow (c). However, because of the multihole configuration of the needle it has gained access to both lesions (a) and (b) in addition to the area of normal marrow.

*Instrumentation**

The construction and design of this instrument is identical to that of the Islam posterior iliac puncture needle but has multiple side holes in addition to the one frontal opening (Figure 25). The 17.5 mm distal portion of the needle has 14 lateral ports, 4 rows of 8 holes in one plane and 3 rows of 6 holes in another. The rows of apertures are 2.5 mm apart and drilled in a spiral fashion to avoid any weakness which would appear if the drilling for any two ports were executed on the same transverse plane. The first row of holes is made 3.0 mm from the end of the bevelled point and the diameter of each hole is approximately 1.0 mm.

---

*This instrument is also available in different sizes (bore diameters) and lengths.

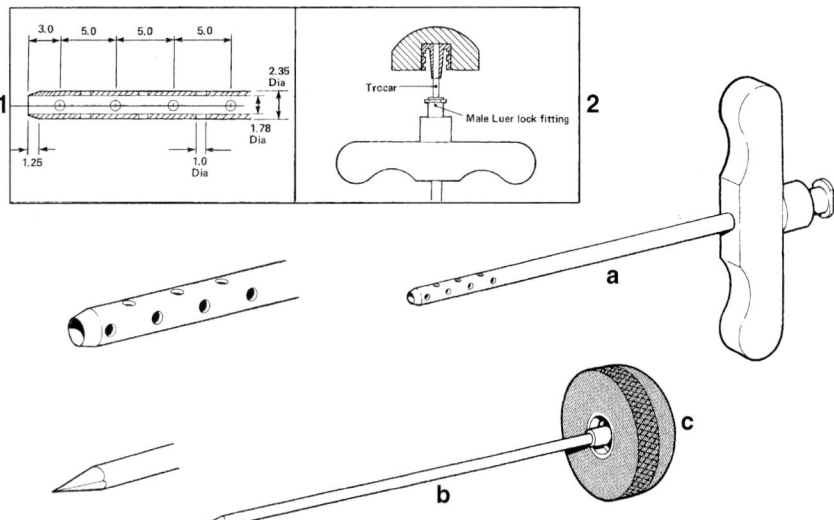

FIGURE 25. The Islam multipore bone marrow aspiration needle. The needle (a), stilette (b) and the handle (c). The inset 1 shows the details of distal 17.5 mm portion of the needle and the inset 2 illustrates the details of the luer lock attachment of the needle and the handle.

Aspiration Procedure

The aspiration procedure with this needle is the same as for any posterior iliac puncture. In this case however, care must be taken to insure that the entire perforated segment of the needle is introduced into the medullary cavity and away from the cortical entry site. This avoids the potential aspiration of air and soft tissue adherent to the externum of the ilium.

PROCESSING OF SPECIMENS

Preparations of Aspirate Smears

Following aspiration of marrow, smears should be made without much delay. This can be done in many several ways. (1) A large drop of marrow with enough fragments can be placed on a slide usually directly from the aspirating needle (Figure 26A) or from the syringe after it has been dislodged from the needle (Figure 26B). Several smears are made by repeatedly collecting the marrow from the slide above and making dry film smear using the edge of the spreader slide as

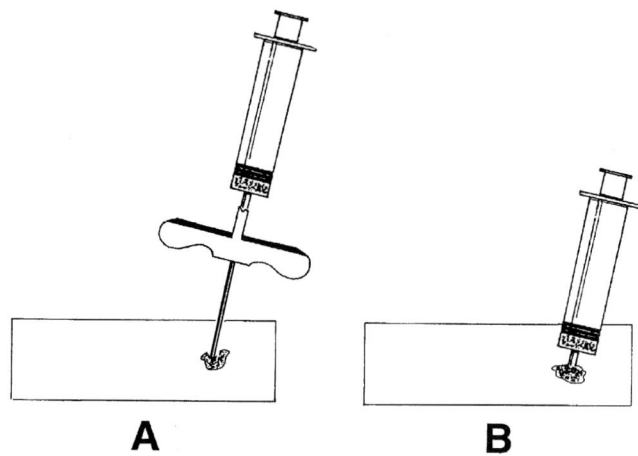

FIGURE 26. Marrow smear preparation. A small amount of aspirated marrow is delivered directly from the aspirating needle (A) or directly from the syringe after it has been dislodged from the needle (B).

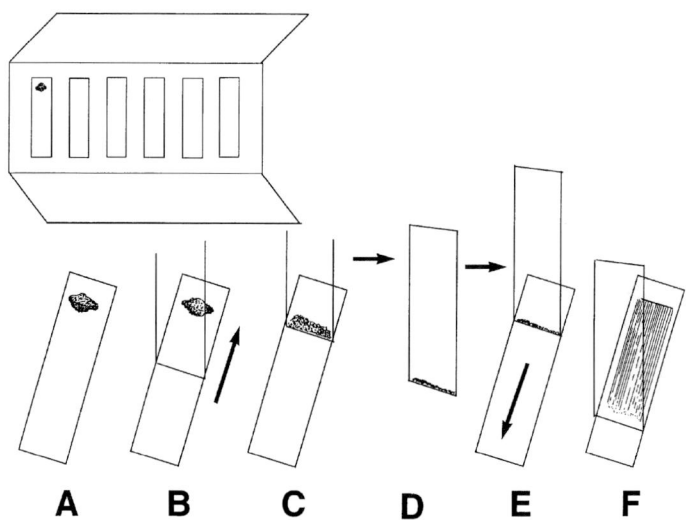

FIGURE 27. An illustration of the method of preparation of several smears from an original sample of marrow by repeatedly collecting the marrow particles with a spreader and making smears using the usual method of smear preparation. (A) Slide with small amount of marrow aspirate, (B) the spreader slide is placed in front of the marrow specimen, (C) the spreader slide is then pulled back towards the marrow sample to collect enough marrow particles at its edge which is then lifted-up (D) and placed on another clean slide (E) and a smear is made. Completed slide (F). The inset shows the arrangement of glass slides for the preparation of such smears. Note that a small amount of marrow is placed at the end of one slide only.

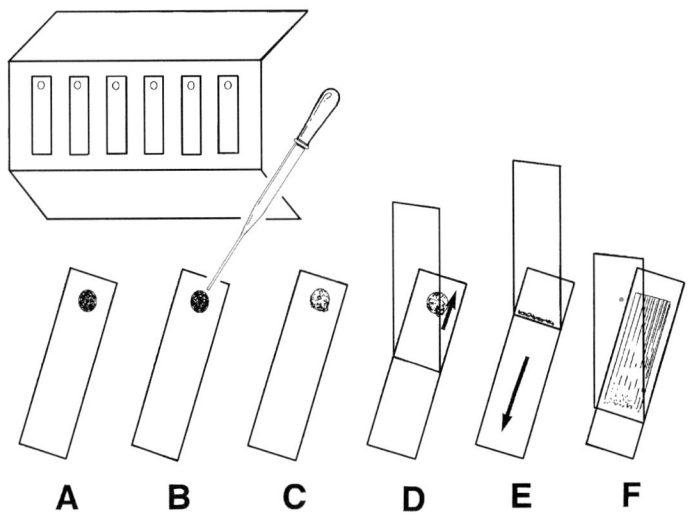

A   B   C   D   E   F

FIGURE 28. An illustration of the method of preparation of marrow smears by placing a drop of marrow aspirate on several glass slides. (A) slide with a small drop of marrow aspirate, (B) excess blood is sucked out with a fine pasteur pipette, (C) slide with the remaining marrow sample containing mostly marrow particles, (D) the spreader slide is pulled back over the remaining marrow sample, (E) spreader slide is advanced in smooth motion, (F) completed slide. The arrangement of the glass slides are shown in the upper left hand corner. Note the drop of marrow on each slide.

shown in Figure 27. (2) Alternatively, a single drop of marrow can be placed on several slides, the excess blood (but not the fragments) is sucked out with a fine pasteur pipette and then smears are made from the remaining samples (Figure 28). (3) A small amount of marrow can be delivered directly into a cuvet (perhaps lined with a non wetable material as teflon or paraffin) containing a suitable anticoagulant. Fragments are then retrieved with a pasteur pipette, delivered on to a slide and smears made in a usual manner (Figure 29). (4) A drop of marrow can be placed in the center of a slide (extra blood may be removed by a fine pasteur pipette) and smears are made by squashing the marrow particles by putting another slide on the top of it and pulling the slides in opposite direction as shown in the illustration (Figure 30). (5) Smears can also be made by putting a drop of marrow or isolated fragments between two cover-slips, and applying slight digital pressure to the "sandwich" and then gently pulling them apart (Figure 31). Some workers routinely add the aspirated marrow to an anticoagulant, e.g. EDTA, in a tube and prepare films at leisure upon return to the laboratory. While this technique is convenient, it requires special care as it is all too easy to use an excessive quantity of the anticoagulant which may then affect the quality of the stained smears. Vacuolization of the cytoplasm and deformation of the nuclei

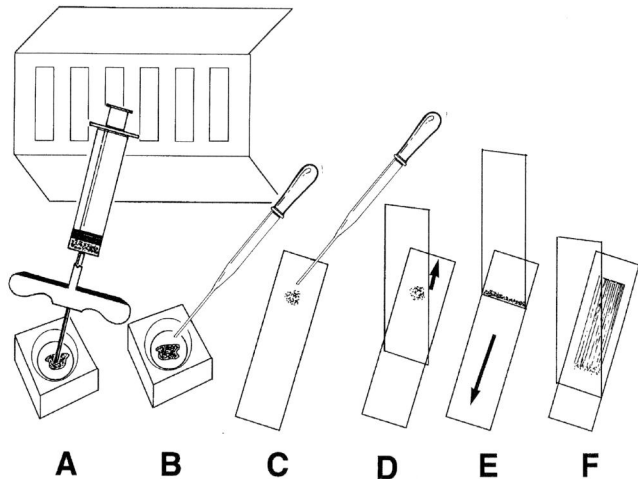

FIGURE 29. Illustration of the method of preparation of marrow smears by first placing a small amount of aspirated marrow into a cuvette containing a suitable anticoagulant. (A) Aspirated marrow being delivered into a cuvette, (B) excess blood (but not the fragments) is sucked out with a fine pasteur pipette and discarded, (C) a drop of marrow sample with the fragments is now withdrawn from the cuvette and placed at one end of a glass slide, (D) the spreader is pulled back over the drop of marrow sample, (E) the spreader slide is gently advanced in smooth motion, (F) completed slide. The cuvettes with marrow sample and the arrangement of slides for the preparation of smears by this method is shown on the left side of the illustration.

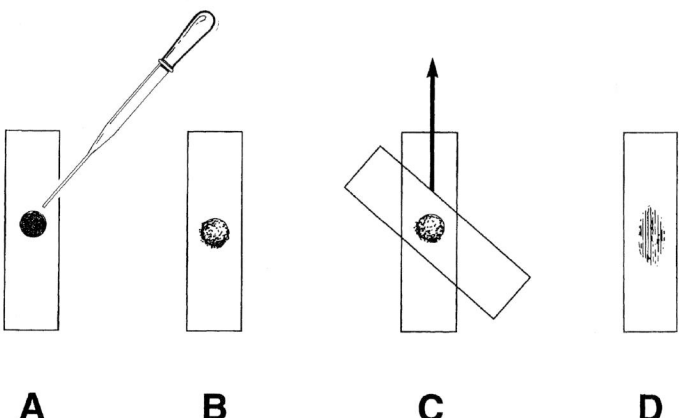

FIGURE 30. Illustration of the method of making squash preparation. (A) A drop of marrow is first placed in the center of a clean glass slide, (B) excess blood is sucked out leaving mostly the marrow particles, (C) another clean glass slide is placed over the marrow fragments and pulled in the direction of the arrow while holding firm the slide with marrow fragments, (D) completed slide.

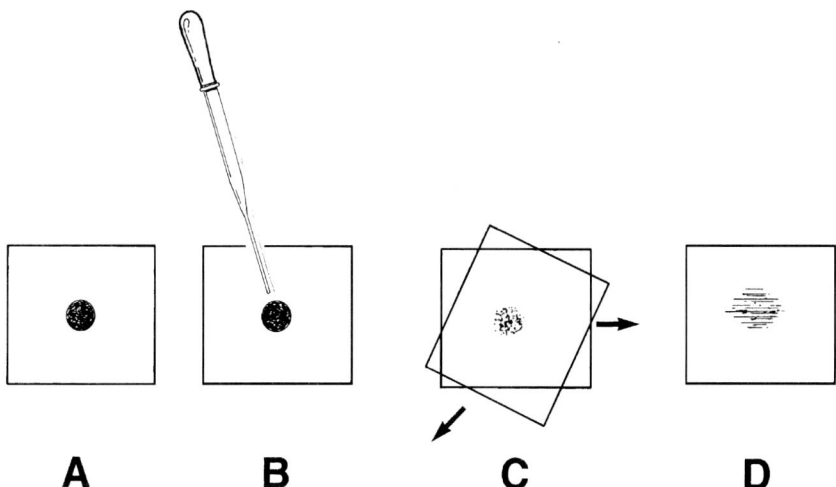

FIGURE 31. Illustration of the coverslip method of making squash preparation. (A) A drop of marrow is placed in the center of a coverslip, (B) excess blood is sucked out with a fine pasteur pipette, (C) a second coverslip is placed over the remaining marrow fragments and the coverslips are pulled in directions of arrows, (D) completed smear (squash).

(e.g. cloverleaf shapes) are also a potential problem if the preparation of the smears is delayed too long. Regardless of the technique of dry film preparation, the smears should be air dried as rapidly as possible to derive the best cytologic presentation. In some circumstances, particularly on days with a high level of humidity, fans can be used to direct a stream of air over the smears or they may be waved in the air to insure rapid drying.

Usually the first or second method of preparation of aspirate smears proves quite satisfactory. It is preferable to select the third method when there is a possibility of rapid clotting of the aspirated marrow as in cases of hypergranular promyelocytic leukaemia. Squashing and smearing of the particles not only causes disruption of the marrow units but also can cause considerable distortion of cells. This technique also tends to produce regionally thick preparations which are difficult to stain well. Although some workers prefer the squash preparations most likely because of prior training and/or long term usage, but this approach has no advantages over the first three described methods. Coverslip preparations require delicate handling because of the fragility of these small thin glass plates. Staining them involves additional work since they are not the dimensions of conventional microscope slides and hence require special holders. They do not readily lend themselves to some automated stainers. They must also be mounted on regular microscope slides after staining to be efficiently examined under a light microscope. Other than the possible advantage of yielding excellent results with minimal sized samples no specific benefits are attributable to this technique.

Concomitant with the preparation of dry film smears, the remainder of the aspirated marrow is delivered into a suitable anticoagulant for flow cytometric and cytogenetic studies and/or into a fixative for the preparation of histological sections. Some of the films should be fixed in absolute methanol as soon as they are dry for staining with one of the Romanowsky type stains (e.g. May-Grunwald-Giemsa, Wright-Giemsa, Leishman) or by the periodic acid Schiff reaction or for marrow iron stores. Additional films should be fixed in formol-ethanol when other cytochemical staining is desired. The staining with the Romanowsky type dyes should be conducted immediately after fixing with methanol.

When no marrow sample is obtained from the aspiration procedure (dry tap) the stilette should be inserted into the needle to push out any material from inside the lumen of the needle on to a slide. This material should be spread into a film and stained. Occassionally in some cases of lymphoma or carcinoma a small but sufficient amount of the malignant tissue is nevertheless drawn into the needle from which a definite diagnosis can be made.

Preparation of Sections from Aspirated Specimens

A number of methods of preparing histologic sections from aspirated fragments of marrow have been published. They all differ to some extent in the details of handling and concentrating the fragments, fixation and embedding. The method described by Lukes and Tindle yields an adequate concentration of the marrow particles and is simple to carry out. It is summarised below.

Method

Following preparation of the smears, and setting aside a portion of the aspirate for flowcytometric and cytogenetic study, the remainder of the marrow (1–3 ml) present in the syringe is expelled into a specimen jar (60 ml) containing 3 ml of EDTA (7 mg/ml) (ethylenediamine tetraacetic acid) for anticoagulation. After thorough mixing, Zenker's fixative solution (half strength) is added, completely filling the container to avoid drying of marrow particles adherent to the sides of the container. Fixation is usually complete within 1–2 minutes. The specimens may be allowed to stand for up to 48 hours without apparent harm using a modified Zenker's solution (FU 48, Technicon Instruments Corp., Tarrytown, N.Y.). The latter does not harden the tissue excessively upon standing, nor does it require washing of the specimen after fixation. The marrow is then filtered through a plastic funnel containing a circular stainless steel foundation mesh No. 120 (United Surgical Supplies Co., Inc., Port Chester, N.Y.) which provides the grid upon which the tissue particles are collected. This filtration technique not only eliminates the erythrocytes but also concentrates the marrow tissue particles. The filtration process may be assisted by negative pressure by placing the funnel with the attached grid on the top of a vacuum bottle. After filtration is complete, the particles on the grid are cautiously lifted off with a scalpel and placed on a clean slide. Fluid is removed with blotting paper applied at the margins of the area of the particles. The marrow particles are aggregated according to the examiner's requirements and covered with a 2% agar suspension previously maintained at 46°C. Upon cooling it forms a tissue mat and holds the particles in place. Sections are cut at 3 to 5 μm in thickness and routinely stained with haematoxylin and eosin (H & E) and/or the periodic acid Schiff method (PAS) with a hematoxylin counterstain. The Prussian blue method is also used to stain and quantitate haemosiderin. The PAS method serves as an excellent differential stain.

Special considerations

The fragments of bone marrow aspirated by puncture technique are typically small (less than 1 mm in diameter) and usually free of bone. As a result the marrow architecture and the relationships that exist between bone and bone marrow cells cannot be studied. In a satisfactory preparation however, the relationship between the haematopoietic and adipose cells is well preserved, hypoplasia or hyperplasia if present can be evaluated, and tumour cells and granulomata can be identified. The usefulness of such sections is limited by their small dimensions making it uncertain how representative they are of the total bone marrow. A more significant disadvantage of histologic sections of aspirated marrow is that when no bone marrow units are obtained, as in some cases of aplasia, myelosclerosis, packed marrow of acute or chronic leukaemia, or replacement by tumor cells, this procedure fails to provide any definitive diagnostic information. A trephine biopsy consequently becomes mandatory when aspiration of the marrow fails to deliver the required tissue. Currently since many haematologists perform bone marrow aspirations at the posterior iliac crest they also simultaneously use the same puncture wound to perform a trephine biopsy, sometimes using the same biopsy needle. As a result the request for histologic sections preparation from aspirated marrow fragments has been reduced considerably. This is quite appropriate since histologic sections of aspirate fragments can not provide the extent of information that is available from histologic sections of a marrow core.

Clinical (bedside) assistance with biopsy procurement

In many hospitals (outpatient department, doctors surgery) haematologists tend to perform the entire bone marrow examination (bone marrow aspiration and bone marrow biopsy) procedure single handedly without the help of an assistant. The entire procedure, as is quite apparent, entails multiple steps some of which require speed, accuracy and clinical skill (e.g preparing the patient, administering the anaesthesia, making the smear etc). Further potential complications are the immediate clotting of the sample in some patients and/or bleeding at the puncture site if the wound is not attended and pressure applied after the needle is withdrawn. Therefore help from an assistant/haematology technician can facilitate the procedure considerably. He or she can stand by the side of the bed, lay out slides on a tray while the haematologist prepares and drapes the patient. He/she can also help the clinician withdraw the local anaesthetic into a syringe and following aspiration can receive the aspirated material, prepare the smears, and transfer the marrow into vials for further tests while the clinician tends to the wound and prepares himself/herself to perform the marrow (core) biopsy procedure. See photograph 1–7 demonstrating the in-clinic bone marrow biopsy procedure.

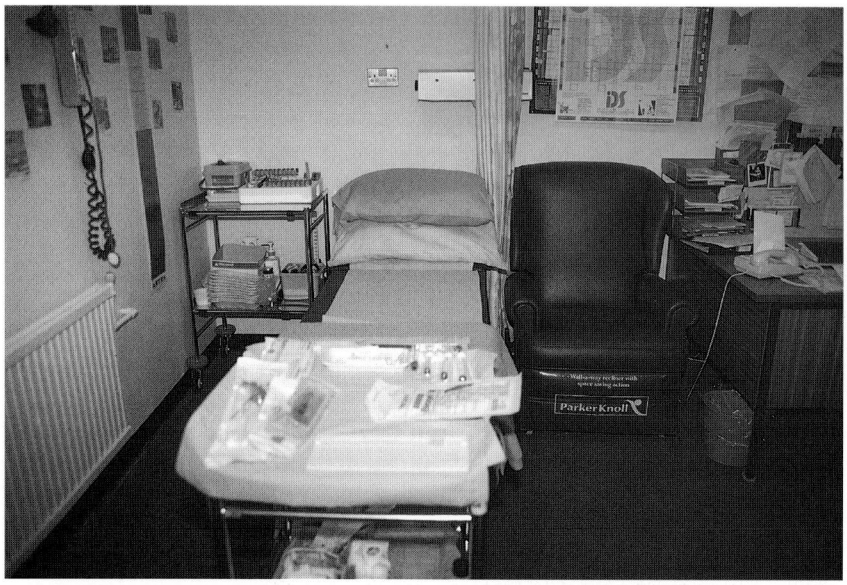

PHOTOGRAPH 1. Note the adjustable bed for the patient placed in a private setting. A technician's tray containing needles syringes, gauze, antiseptic, bone marrow aspiration and biopsy needles etc is placed adjacent to the bed.

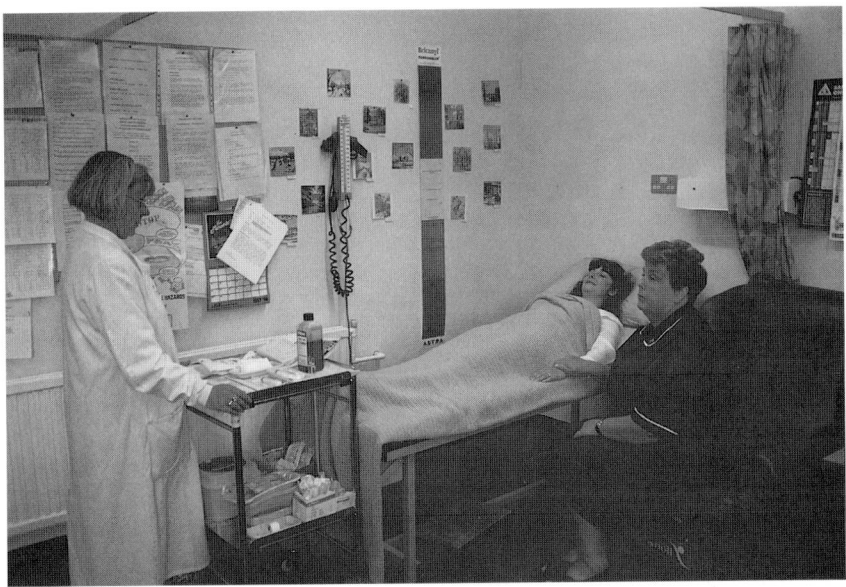

PHOTOGRAPH 2. Shows a patient lying in the bed, a technician who will assist in the process standing in front of the tray and the sister in charge (holding the hand of the patient).

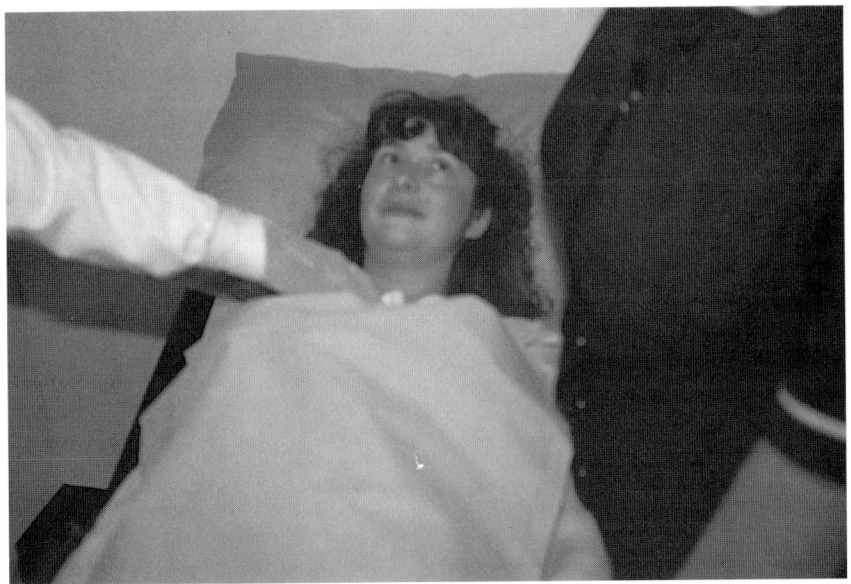

PHOTOGRAPH 3. Shows tending of the wound by the operator. Pressure is being applied with the left hand to the sternal bone marrow aspiration site.

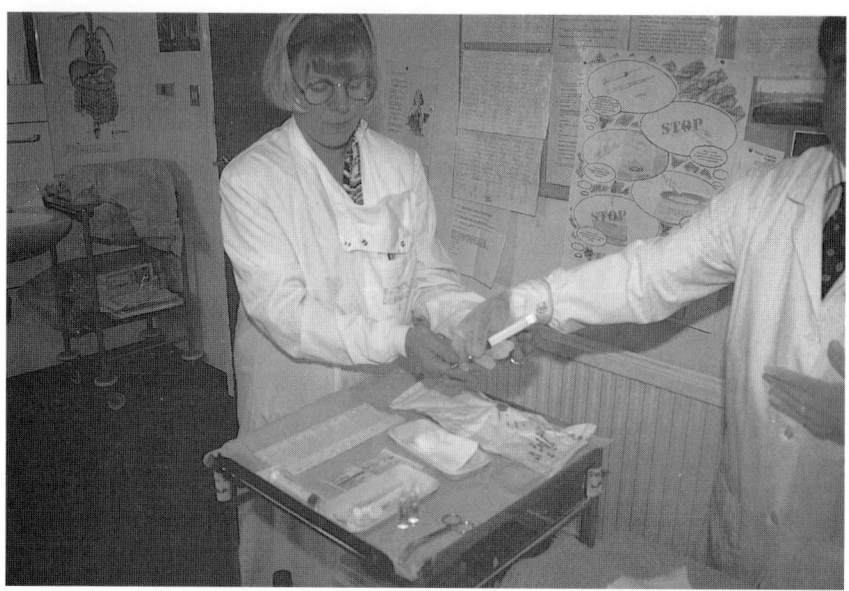

PHOTOGRAPH 4. Shows delivery of the aspirated marrow to the technician for the preparation of smears and utilization of the remainder of the marrow for other uses.

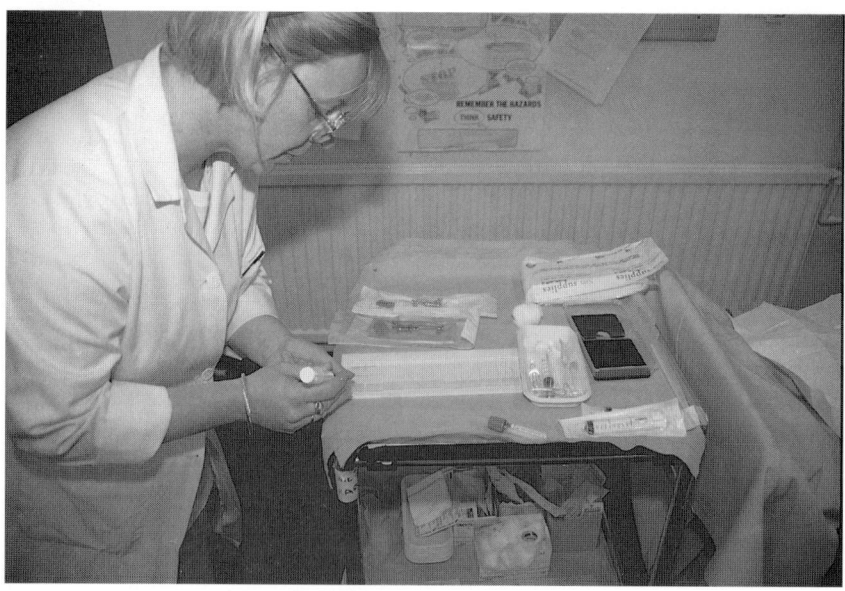

PHOTOGRAPH 5. Shows careful preparation of the smears by the technician.

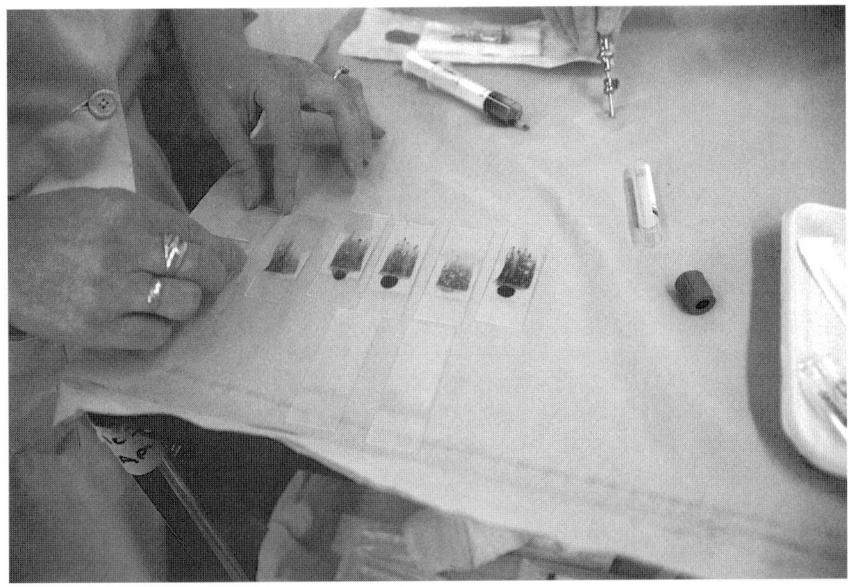

PHOTOGRAPH 6. Shows careful preparation of the smears by the technician.

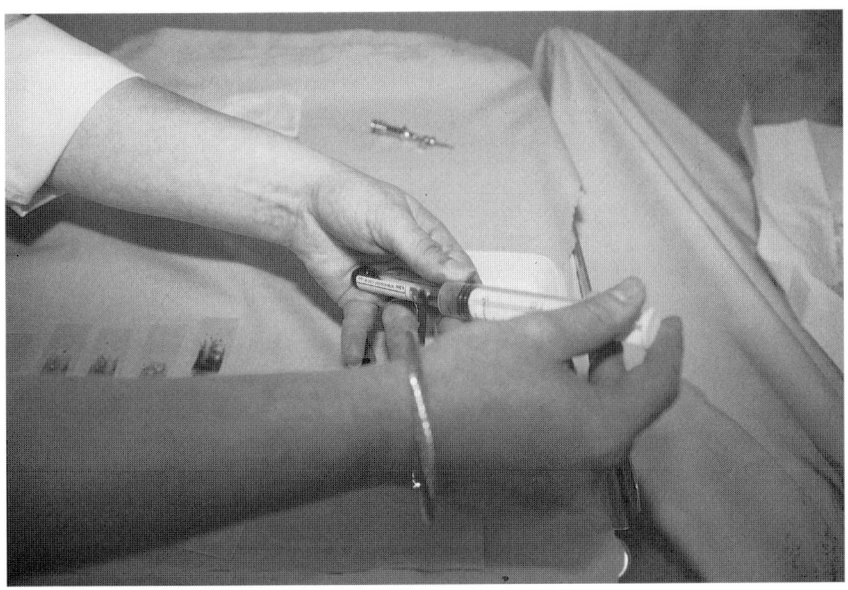

PHOTOGRAPH 7. Shows residual marrow being delivered into a bottle containing sequestrene for additional uses.

METHODS OF STAINING SMEARS

The films are first dried in air (rapidly), then fixed by immersing the slides in a Coplin jar containing absolute methanol for 5–10 minutes. They are then transfered (according to one well recognised technique) to a staining jar containing May-Grunwald stain freshly diluted with an equal volume of Sorensen's phosphate buffer pH 6.8 and filtered through a Whatman filter paper No. 1. After the films have been allowed to stain for 15–20 minutes, they are then immediately transfered (without washing) to another jar containing Giemsa stain freshly diluted with 9 volumes of Sorensen's phosphate buffer pH 6.8 and filtered through a No.1 Whatman filter paper. After staining in the Giemsa stain for 10–15 minutes, the slides are dipped ("washed") several times in Sorensen's phosphate buffer pH 6.8 and then allowed to stand undisturbed in water for 2–5 minutes for differentiation to take place. This may be controlled by inspection of the wet slide under the low power of the miscroscope; with experience the colour of the film as observed by the naked-eye is often a good guide. During staining the slides should be transfered from one staining solution to the other without being allowed to dry. The intensity of the staining is also affected by any variation in the thickness of a film and as a result it is often not easy to obtain uniform staining throughout a film's length. This is the rationale for excercising care in selecting the proper region (where morphology and staining characteristics of marrow cells are at their best) of a smear for morphologic assessment.

After staining the smears are airdried and mounted with a cover-glass using diatex or permount as the mounting medium. The coverslip prevents the film becoming scratched during subsequent handling and also facilitates microscopy at less than oil immersion magnifications. However if desirable the slides need not be coverslipped. They can be examined under immersion oil which can be removed by gently wiping the slide with tissue or dipping it into xylol. Such films will retain their usefulness and will not deteriorate for an indefinite period.

Most laboratories presently use automated staining machines (Figure 32) and if properly employed they provide good quality staining for both peripheral blood and bone marrow films. However, smears containing obvious, readily recognizable bone marrow fragments are more likely to loose these structures when stained by machine rather than the more gentle staining in a Coplin jar or by the flooding method. Bone marrow smears should also be routinely stained by Perl's reaction (Prussian blue technique) to evaluate non-haem iron stores (haemosiderin, ferritin) and to establish the presence or absence of sideroblasts.

EXAMINATION OF SMEARS

Careful preparation of films from aspirated marrow is essential. The haematologist's dependence on good staining to derive a correct interpretation of a marrow smear cannot be over emphasized. A preparation can be considered satisfactory

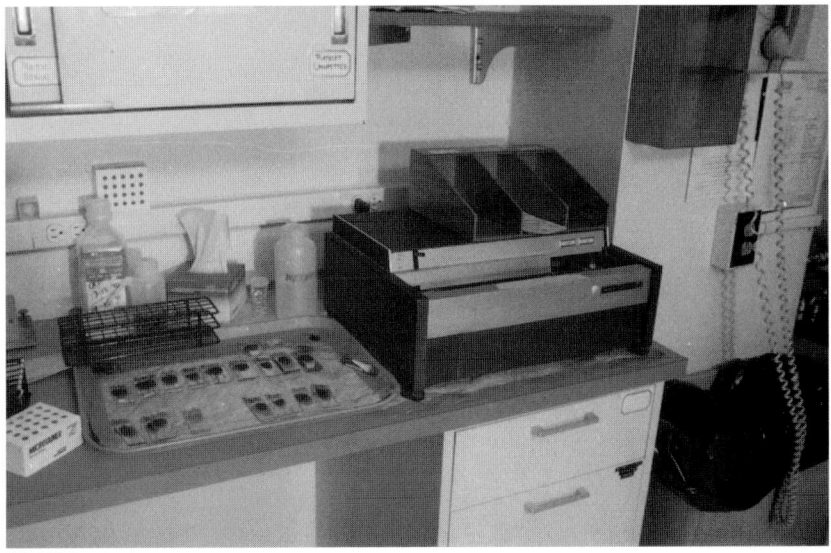

FIGURE 32. An automated staining machine.

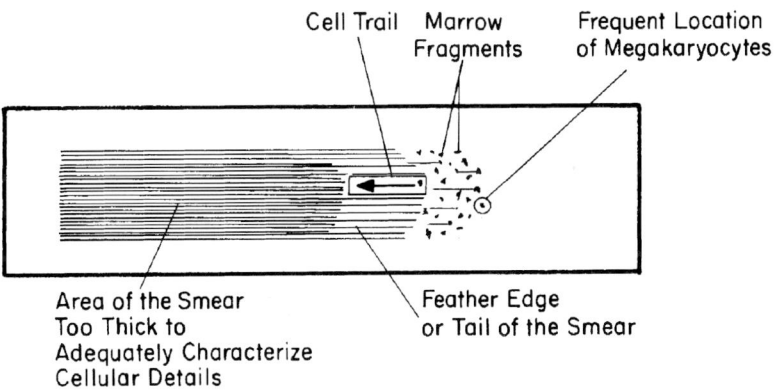

Cell Trail   Marrow   Frequent Location
             Fragments   of Megakaryocytes

Area of the Smear
Too Thick to
Adequately Characterize
Cellular Details

Feather Edge
or Tail of the Smear

FIGURE 33. Schematic drawing of a bone marrow aspirate smear. The smear has been spread from left to right.

only when an adequate number of marrow particles as well as enough free marrow cells are present (Figure 33). In order to effectively analyze an aspirate at least two or more slides should be examined. The initial reading should begin with an overall assessment of the marrow film with an examination under low power (10x objective). This insures that large cells as megakaryocytes, osteoclasts, clusters or aggregates of metastatic cells or macrophages or even erythroblastic islets will not be missed or overlooked because of an inadequate survey.

The differential counts should be made in the trails of cells commencing from a marrow fragment in the distal end (feather edge) of the smear and working back towards the head (beginning) of the film (Figure 33). The morphology of haematopoietic cells that are close to the fragments from which they originated is most likely to be optimal. Cells that are more distal or near to the origin of the smear reside in the thicker region of the film and are less likely to be morphologically ideal. Trails of several marrow fragments in one or several bone marrow aspirate smears should be examined to make an adequate reading. Megakaryocytes are often dragged along with the fragments. Consequently before reporting that megakaryocytes are either reduced or absent areas close to the marrow fragments should be thoroughly examined and searched for their presence.

REPORTING AND INTERPRETATION

The reporting of a bone marrow should begin with an analysis of the marrow particles to assess the marrow cellularity. The degree of cellularity can be assessed within broad limits as increased, normal or decreased by careful inspection of several marrow fragments in one or more stained films. The bone marrow is considered normocellular when the volumetric ratio between haematopoietic cells and fat is about 50%/50%. The cellularity of the marrow is affected by age and this physiological variation has to be taken into account in one's evaluation of the tissue. In adults, a relatively smaller portion of the marrow cavity is occupied by haemopoietic marrow than in children and the proportion of fat cells to active marrow is increased. In subjects aged 60 or more the marrow tends to become still more fatty; this is particularly true for the manubrium sterni. It is known that the marrow undergoes slight to moderate hyperplasia in pregnancy.

Following assesment of the cellularity the evaluation of the bone marrow should address the qualitative and quantitative aspects of erythropoiesis, granulopoiesis, thrombopoiesis and the presence or absence of any abnormal cells. This is ideally done in the cell trails. Megakaryocytes are most visible near the fragments. Then an assesment of iron stores and presence or absence of ring sideroblasts should be made. Finally a comment should be made as to the reviewer's overall impression of the marrow.

An Effective, Useful Bone Marrow Report Should Comment on the Following

1. **Site**: bone marrow aspirate obtained from the sternum, right or left posterior iliac crest etc, under local anaesthesia.
2. **Overall cellularity**: normal, increased or decreased. The increase or decrease can further be qualified by a prefix as either mild, moderate or marked. Bone marrow cellularity can not be adequately assessed if few or no fragments are available in the aspirate.

3. **Erythropoiesis**: activity – normal, increased or decreased; matuaration sequence (normoblastic vs megaloblastic); cytologic abnormalities such as dyserythropoietic changes, etc.

4. **Granulopoiesis**: activity – normal, increased or decreased; maturation sequence (i.e. whether all stages of maturation are represented or if there is a maturation arrest); cytologic abnormalities such as dysgranulopoiesis (giant metamyelocytes, Pelger-Huet forms etc.); the presence and number of myeloblasts and promyelocytes.

5. **Megakaryopoiesis**: numerical assesment (increased, normal or decreased); maturation sequence, platelet production, pleomorphism; cytologic abnormalities such as dysmegakaryopoiesis (multinucleated forms etc.).

6. **Plasma cell series**: numerical assessment (expressed in percentage), maturation, inclusion bodies, any abnormalities or neoplastic changes.

7. **Lymphocyte series**: lymphoid aggregates, germinal centers, numerical assessment (expressed in percentage), morphologic abnormalities (large, small, cleaved, character of nucleoli), malignancies.

8. **Eosinophils and basophils**: numerical assessment (expressed in percentage), any abnormalities.

9. **Iron stores**: content (normal, increased or decreased), the presence or absence of ring sideroblasts.

10. **Miscellaneous**: presence of macrophages, mast cells, granulomas, amyloidosis, gelatinous transformation of fat, pathologic lesions of the bone, osteoblasts, osteoclasts and metastic neoplasms etc.

11. **Differential cell count**: a detailed differential count (**myelogram**) is not always necessary but sometimes they may be useful. The normal ranges for differential counts on aspirated bone marrow are given in Table 1.

12. **Comment/conclusion**: overall impression of the marrow as being normal or abnormal. If abnormal – identify the abnormality, any further investigations such as vit. B12 and/or folic acid assays for megaloblastic anaemias; serum iron, TIBC etc. for iron deficiency anaemia and any other studies that are recommended to be performed.

COMMON PROBLEMS AND THEIR RESOLUTION

Although a satisfactory sample of bone marrow can be aspirated without much difficulty from the sternum or from the posterior iliac crest (the most commonly used sites), occasionally it may be necessary to re-insert the stilette and advance the needle a little further or to reinsert the needle into the bone in a slightly different position in order to access the tissue. Sometimes, however, no marrow can be aspirated resulting in a dry tap. In such circumstances the stilette, as indicated previously should be inserted into the needle to push out any material within the lumen of the needle on to a slide to examine the tissue lodged therein.

TABLE 1. Normal ranges for differential counts on aspirated bone marrow

Reticulum cells	0.1–2%
Myeloblasts	0.1–3%
Neutrophil promyelocytes	0.1–5%
Neutrophil myelo and metamyelocytes	17–41%
Neutrophil bands and segmented form	15–32%
Eosinophils and precursors	1–5%
Basophils and precursors	0–1%
Monocytes	0–4%
Lymphocytes	7–23%
Plasma cells	0.1–3.5%
Proerythroblasts	0.1–2%
Basophilic erythroblasts	0.1–4%
Polychromatophilic erythroblasts	5–20%
Orthochromatic erythroblasts	2–10%
Myeloid/erythroid ratio	2.5–10:1

An optimal myelogram requires the enumeration of a minimum of 200–500 cells.

Needle Breakage During Aspiration Procedure

Rarely, a bone marrow aspiration needle (particularly of the older generation of Salah or Klima type needles when they are used for posterior iliac crest aspiration) may break while being inserted into or withdrawn from the bone. In such circumstances an attempt should be made to keep the distal broken portion of the needle exposed and always in view of the operator (that is to keep the needle visible and avoiding the possibility of its loss in a mass of depressed and then rebounded soft tissue mass). This is accomplished by pressing the tissue surrounding the needle with fingers of the left hand while trying to clamp or secure the needle with a needle holder. Haemostats like artery forceps are usually unsatisfactory for this purpose. Once the needle is secured it is then removed by gentle alternating rotary motion of the needle holder. If however, for some reason the broken needle is retained within the flesh then the patient should be reassuringly informed of the mishap, the site of the aspiration properly marked, a roentgenogram obtained, and a surgeon notified for consultation.

SELECTED READING

Bennike, T., Gormsen, H. and Moller, B. (1956) Comparative studies of bone marrow punctures of the sternum, the iliac crest and the spinous process. *Acta Medica. Scand.*, **155**, 377–396.

Dacie, J.V. and Lewis, S.M. (1995) *Practical Haematology*. Churchill Livingstone, London, New York.

Emery, J.L. (1957) The technique of bone marrow aspiration in children. *J. Clin. Pathol.*, **10**, 339–341.

Engeset, A., Nesheim, A. and Sokolowski, J. (1979) Incidence of dry tap on bone marrow aspirations in lymphomas and carcinomas: Diagnostic value of the small material in the needle. *Scand. J. Haematol.*, **22**, 417–422.

Gruppo, R.A., Lampkin, B.C. and Granger, S. (1977) Bone marrow cellularity determination: Comparison of the biopsy, aspirate and buffy coat. *Blood*, **49**, 29–36.

Hyun, B.H. (1988) Hematology/Oncology Clinics of North America, *Bone Marrow Examination*, **2**(40).

Islam, A. (1983) A new bone marrow aspiration needle to overcome the sampling errors inherent in the technique of bone marrow aspiration. *J. Clin. Pathol.*, **36**, 954–958.

Islam, A. (1991) A new sternal puncture needle. *J. Clin. Pathol.*, **44**, 690–691.

Knowles, S. and Hoffbrand, A.V. (1980) Bone marrow aspiration and biopsy. *Br. Med. J.*, **281**, 204–205.

Loge, J.P. (1948) Spinous process puncture. A simple clinical approach for obtaining bone marrow. *Blood*, **3** 198–???

Lukes, R.J. and Tindle, B.H. (1972) An approach to bone marrow evaluation by pathologists. *Anatomic and Clinical Pathology*, **Series No. 285**, 86–92.

Prasad, R. and Olsen, W.H. (1987) Bone marking for biopsy using radionuclide bone imaging. *Cancer*, **60**, 2205–2207.

CHAPTER 3

BONE MARROW TREPHINE BIOPSY

INTRODUCTION

The technique of bone marrow biopsy was first introduced by Ghedini of Genoa in 1908 when he performed a surgical bone marrow biopsy on a patient to aid in the diagnosis of a haematologic disease. He obtained a sample of bone and marrow from the upper end of the tibia of an adult using a manual trephine. Although the value of bone marrow biopsy in the diagnosis of bone and bone marrow disorders have long been recognised, it is only fairly recently that the technique has become popular and gained some acceptance among haematologists and oncologists. This is specifically due to two reasons; (1) development of new needles ensuring that the biopsies can be carried out with virtually no discomfort to the patient while imposing little or no damage to the biopsied tissue (Figure 34), and (2) improvements in the technique of processing bone marrow biopsies in plastic (methyl and glycol-methacrylate) which require no decalcification. This approach provides thin (1–2 μm) sections of high histological quality that are stainable with Romanowsky type stains (Giemsa or May-Grunwald & Giemsa) providing excellent cytomorphologic detail of the haemopoietic tissue (Figure 35a&b). It has also become apparent that much more diagnostic and prognostic information can be obtained from adequately processed and properly stained bone marrow biopsy sections than from dry film smears alone.

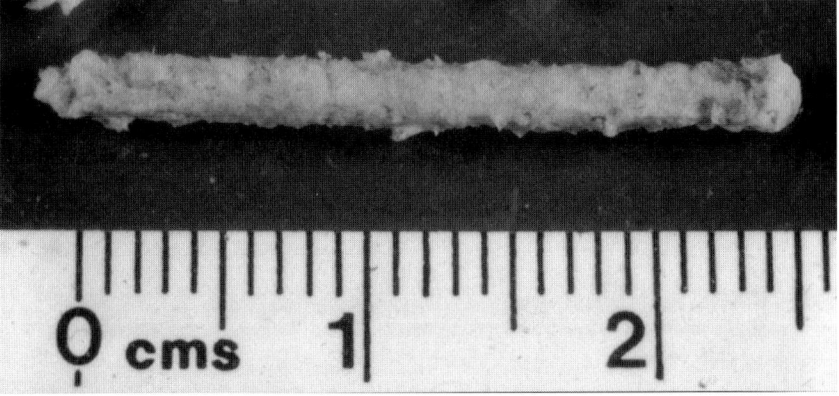

FIGURE 34. A bone marrow biopsy specimen obtained from the right posterior iliac crest using a (standard size) Islam bone marrow biopsy needle. Note the long and uniform core of marrow tissue obtained by the procedure.

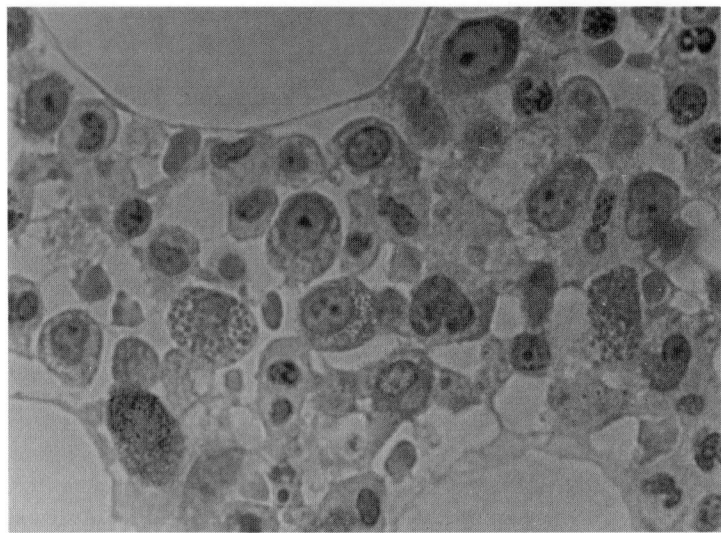

FIGURE 35a. Bone marrow biopsy section from a normal adult showing elements of granulopoiesis. Note a myeloblast, two eosiniphilic granulocytes, a basophil granulocyte, a few neutrophilic myelocytes and their segmented forms. (The section was processed in methyl-methacrylate (MMA) and stained with May-Grunwald-Giemsa stain).

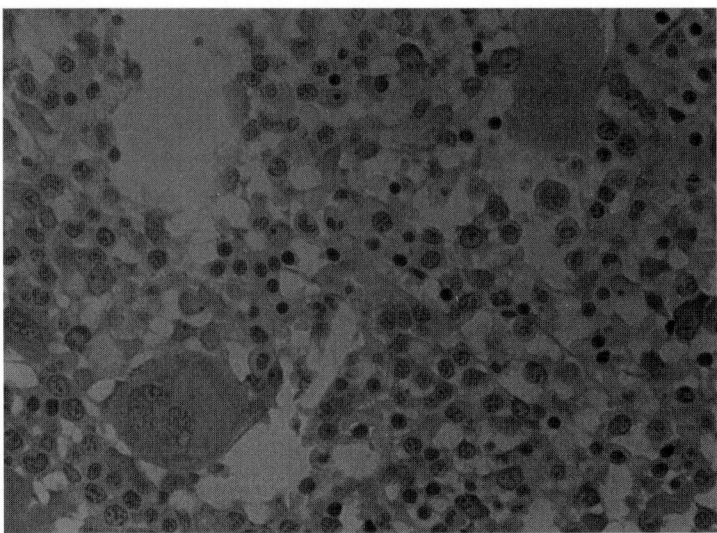

FIGURE 35b. Bone marrow biopsy section from a normal adult showing elements of erythropoiesis in different stages of maturation. Two megakaryocytes and a mast cell are also present. (The section was processed in MMA and stained with May-Grunwald-Giemsa stain).

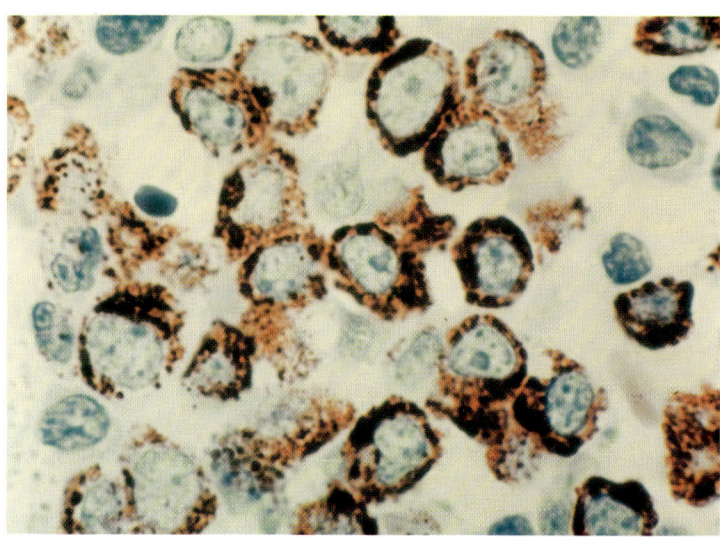

FIGURE 36a. Bone marrow biopsy section from a patient with acute myeloid leukaemia showing myeloperoxidase-positive blast cells. The specimen was processed into glycol-methacrylate (GMA) and stained for myeloperoxidase by Hanker's method.

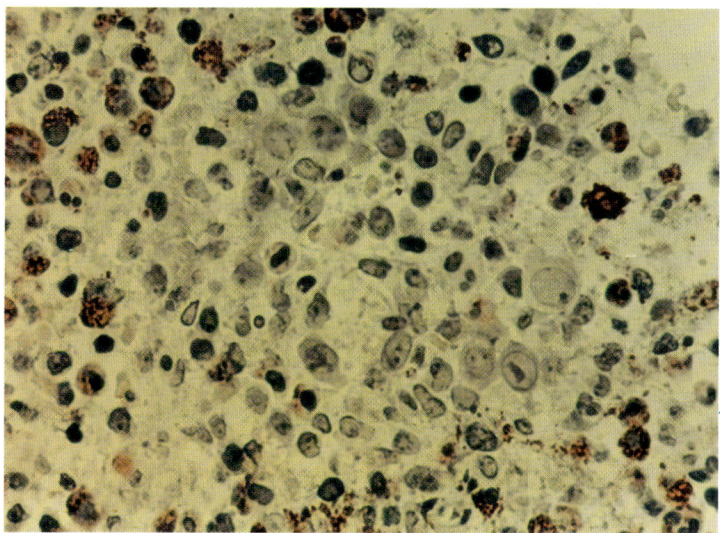

FIGURE 36b. Bone marrow biopsy section from a patient with CML in lymphoblastic transformation. It presents a cluster of myeloperoxidase-negative blast cells. Note the peroxidase positive mature granulocytic cells at the periphery of the lesion. The specimen was processed into GMA and stained for myeloperoxidase by Hanker's method.

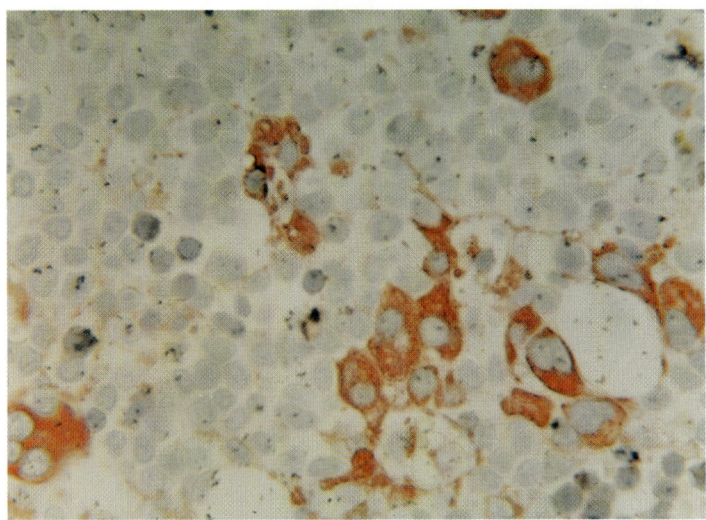

FIGURE 36c. Bone marrow biopsy preparation from a patient with chronic granulocytic leukaemia in megakaryoblastic transformation. The section was stained for factor VIII- related antigen with an indirect immunoperoxidase method and counterstained with Mayer's haematoxylin. The reaction product was demonstrated by using AEC as substrate. Note the strong positive reaction throughout the cytoplasm of the megakaryocytes including the megakaryoblasts.

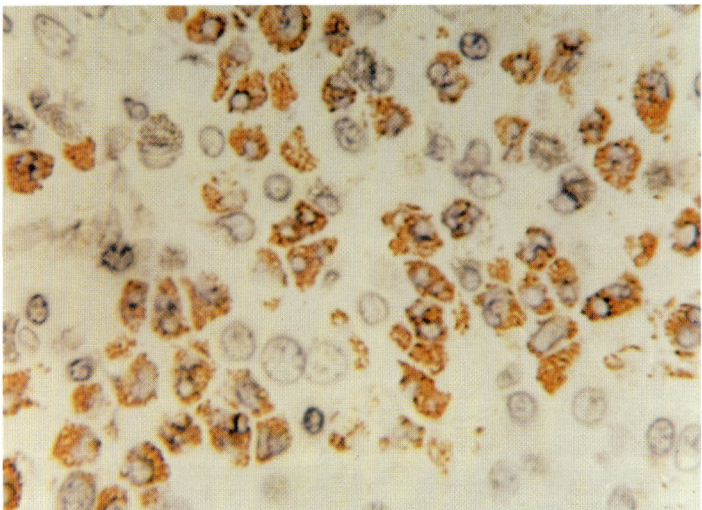

FIGURE 36d. Bone marrow biopsy preparation from a patient with chronic granulocytic leukaemia in chronic phase. The section was stained with monoclonal antibody L12-2 (a marker for mature granulocytes) with an indirect immunoperoxidase method and counterstained with Mayer's haematoxylin. The reaction product was shown by using AEC as substrate. Note strong positive reaction for L12-2 among all mature granulocytic cells.

The ability to perform enzymatic and immunohistological analyses on decalcified (paraffin-embedded) and undecalcified (plastic-embedded) bone marrow biopsies (Figure 36a-d) has added additional impetus and new dimensions to the diagnostic evaluation of bone marrow.

Furthermore, the molecular genetic techniques, such as *in situ* mRNA hybridization, interphase cytogenetics and PCR amplification of DNA for evaluation of minimal residual leukaemia/lymphoma in bone marrow biopsies are opening new frontiers in the diagnostic and aetiologic evaluation of bone marrow biopsies in haematologic and non-haematologic malignant conditions. These techniques are particularly useful in cases where attempts at aspirating bone marrow fails and no malignant cells are available from peripheral blood (for example in certain leukaemias with densely packed marrow or marrows associated with considerable fibrosis and peripheral pancytopenia).

Traditionally bone marrow has been examined in Romanowsky stained smears of aspirated marrow. Although such preparations provide excellent cytomorphologic details of haemopoietic tissue, they are unable to detect, in most instances, focal pathological lesions that may be present in the bone marrow. They are also unsatisfactory in cases of inadequate, unsatisfactory or failed aspirations. In addition they do not reveal any characteristic or spatial localization of particular cell types [such as abnormal localization of immature precursors (ALIP's) in myelodysplastic syndromes and paratrabecular clustering of immature myeloid precursors observed in the accelerated and blastic phase of chronic myeloid leukaemia] and structural and vascular histologic organization of the marrow.

Bone marrow biopsy on the other hand not only overcomes most (if not all) of the disadvantages associated with bone marrow aspiration while in addition sections of the tissue thus obtained can be studied as an organ with its architecture and cellular components both presented in their own natural environment. A bone marrow biopsy thus offers a broader basis for the comprehension of marrow function in health and in disease.

Site(s)

As in bone marrow aspiration, bone marrow biopsies can also be obtained from many different sites. A satisfactory sample of marrow core can be obtained from the anterior or posterior iliac crest. Other sites such as ribs, vertebral bodies, tibia, femur, humerus, ischial tuberosity etc. can also be used. These additional sites for bone marrow biopsy are used only in the presence of radiologic or other evidence of osseus lesions to obtain diagnostic material.

At present most bone marrow biopsies are performed at the posterior iliac crest. This is because of the advent of newer needles which are easier to manipulate and thereby making their access to the posterior iliac crest much easier. In most instances an adequate biopsy sample can be obtained from this site. The bone of the anterior iliac crest, however, is too thick and is difficult to penetrate with standard bone marrow biopsy needles. It is possible to obtain satisfactory specimens from this locus with manually operated boring trephines and electric drills but they require an open surgical procedure, and in most instances, the procedure cannot be repeated on the same site for at least 4–6 months. Conversely, the posterior iliac crest is comparatively less dense than the anterior iliac crest and presents the largest readily accessible area of marrow-rich bone in the body. This area is also distant from any vital structure thus serious accidents or complications are unlikely. With brief training and minimal experience biopsies of adequate size can be easily obtained from this site with an appropriate bone marrow biopsy needle. More importantly perhaps, this region can be re-biopsied as often as every four to six weeks as required for monitoring the marrow following chemotherapy or other therapeutic modalities.

Method

There are several different ways that a bone marrow biopsy sample can be obtained e.g. by an open surgical biopsy, with electric myelotomy drills, with manually operated boring trephines, and with bone marrow biopsy needles. Each technique has its limitations, advantages and disadvantages.

Open surgical biopsy

The sole advantage of an open surgical marrow biopsy is that it allows a larger segment of bone and marrow to be obtained and examined. This method on the other hand has several disadvantages. It has to be carried out in an operating theatre under general anaesthesia and with full aseptic procedure. It may be risky if the patient has a bleeding disorder or granulocytopenia, while in leukaemic patients the incision may fail to heal. One of the significant drawbacks of an open surgical biopsy is that the procedure can seldom be repeated at the same site. Surgical bone marrow biopsy is rarely, if ever, required in haematological problems.

Electric myelotomy drill (Figure 37)

This technique was pioneered by Rolf Burkhardt of Munich, Germany in the 1970's. This is the superior (or vertical) approach for an iliac crest biopsy (Figure 38). In this technique the patient lies in the supine position and the anterior iliac crest area is prepared; 10 to 15 ml of 1% lignocane is used to anaesthetise the skin, subcutaneous tissue and periosteum. A 1 to 2 cm long incision is made directly over the border of the iliac crest, about 2 to 3 cm posterior to the anterior superior iliac spine (Figure 39a). The guide funnel is introduced through the incision by a to and fro twist around its vertical axis until it touches the periosteum. An assistant then holds the funnel which is anchored to the periosteum by pressure leverage of its sharp-toothed lower end. The punch is introduced through the funnel, the tissues are cut circularly at the base of the funnel by rotating the handle

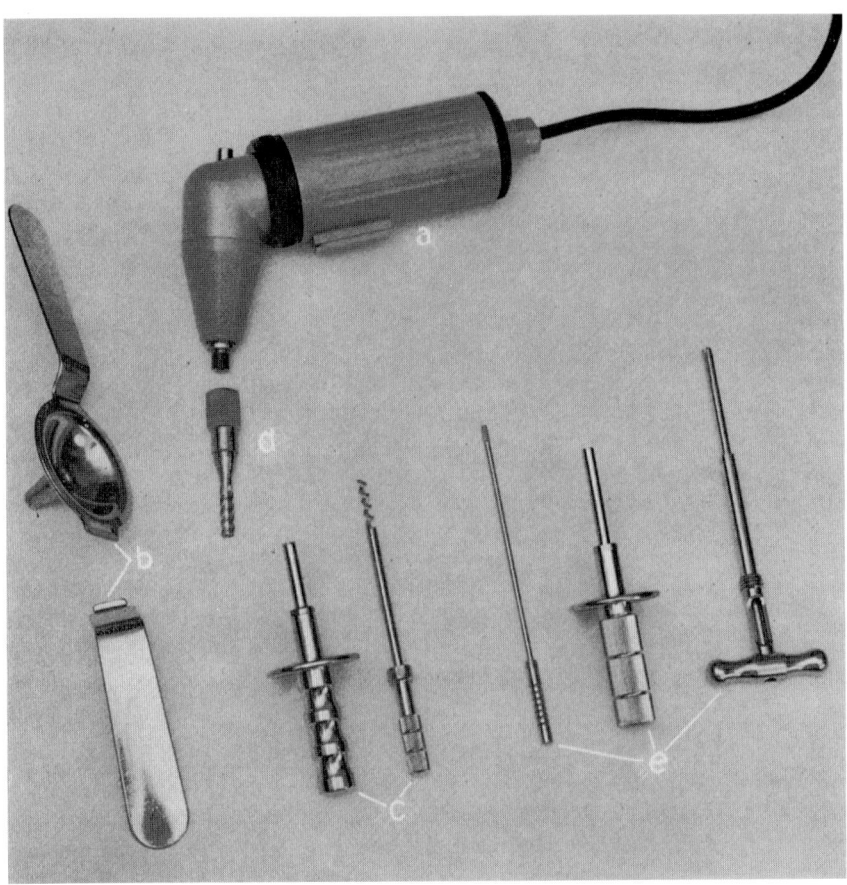

FIGURE 37. Components of Burkhardt's electric myelotomy drill. (a) Low voltage drive motor and gearing in sterilizable casing. (b) Guide funnel with lower sharp-toothed edge. (c) Punch for the removal of tissue external to the periosteum (disassembled). (d) Concave cutter with sharp-toothed, slightly inward-drawn, edge and spiral cutting grooves on the outside. (e) Pincers with spring leaves to appose their free ends by counter rotating the outer sleeve, which is conically narrowed at the bottom. The interior contains an ejector pin (disassembled). (Reproduced from *Bone Marrow and Bone Tissue: Color Atlas of Clinical Histopathology* by Rolf Burkhardt (1971), Springer-Verlag, New York, Heidelberg, Berlin.)

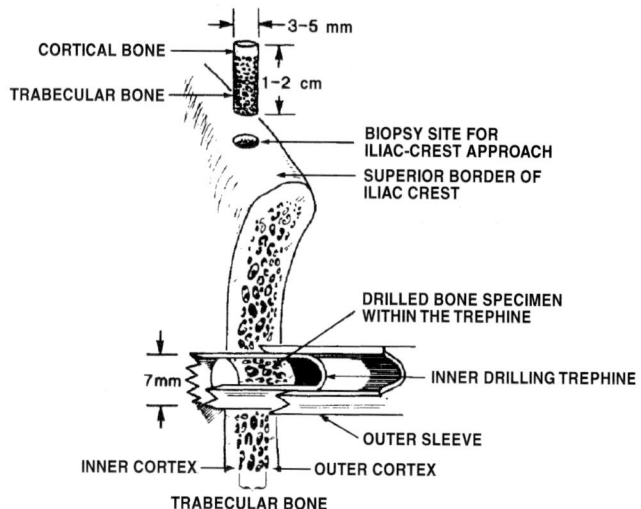

FIGURE 38. Details of two [vertical (superior) and horizontal (transiliac)] types of iliac bone marrow biopsies. (Reproduced from *Bone Histomorphometry: Techniques and Interpretation* by Robert R. Recker (1983), CRC Press, Inc, Boca Raton, Florida.)

within the punch. Soft tissue remnants and blood are cleaned from the periosteum with splinter forceps and swab. The motor driven cutter (electric myelotomy drill) is then introduced along the funnel until it touches the pelvic wing in a longitudinal direction (Figure 39b). Once an adequate length of marrow is cored, the cutter is withdrawn and the pincers are gently inserted over the reamed tissue cylinder. The leaves of the pincers are closed by gently turning the sleeve, and they are levered out by a short pull after two lateral movements. The leaves of the pincers are opened and the biopsy sample is extruded out by the ejector pin (Figure 39c). A Topostasin stick is placed in the opening of the bone for haemostasis, the skin is sutured and the wound dressed with a gauze swab. An elastic pressure bandage is placed around the pelvis which remains for 24 hours during which period the patient is advised to stay in bed.

Although the preservation of trabecular architecture is usually better with the electric myelotomy drill than with an ordinary trephine needle but this procedure is more invasive, complicated, and requires an assistant. Here, again above all, the technique can not be repeated on the same site for at least 4–6 months. There are also two other problems in the use of electric drills; first, in the use of electric drills there may be an accumulation of 'bone powder' in the periphery of the spongy bone if pressure is exerted during the drilling, and secondly, heat artefacts of bone cells may appear if the speed of the instrument is too high. Thus, experience, care and skill are necessary on the part of the physician while using the instrument to avoid trabecular and cellular damage.

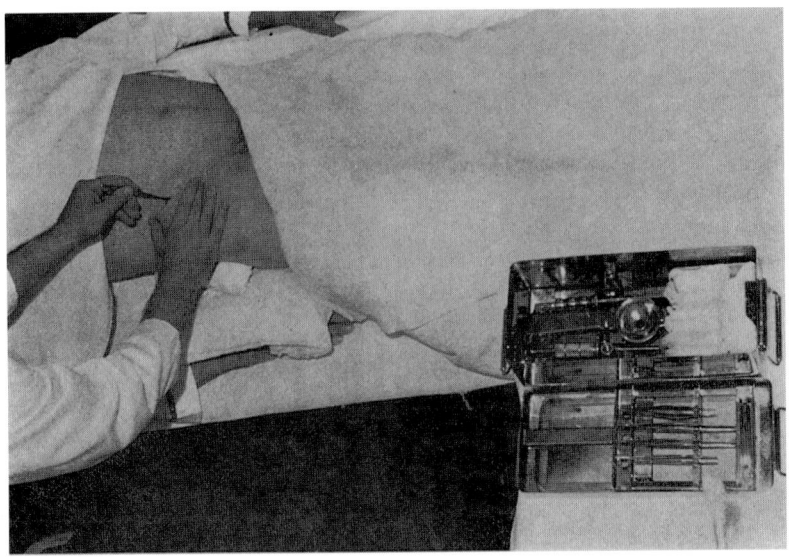

FIGURE 39a. The Burkhardts procedure. Shows an incision being made directly over the iliac crest border. (Reproduced from *Bone Marrow and Bone Tissue: Color Atlas of Clinical Histopathology* by Rolf Burkhardt (1971), Springer-Verlag, New York, Heidelberg, Berlin.)

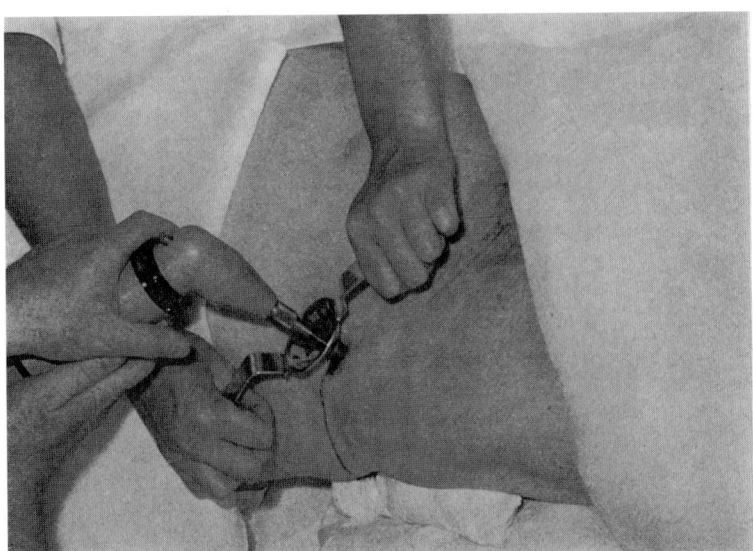

FIGURE 39b. Illustrates the holding of the funnel by an assistant and introduction of the motor driven drill along the funnel. (Reproduced from *Bone Marrow and Bone Tissue: Color Atlas of Clinical Histopathology* by Rolf Burkhardt (1971), Springer-Verlag, New York, Heidelberg, Berlin.)

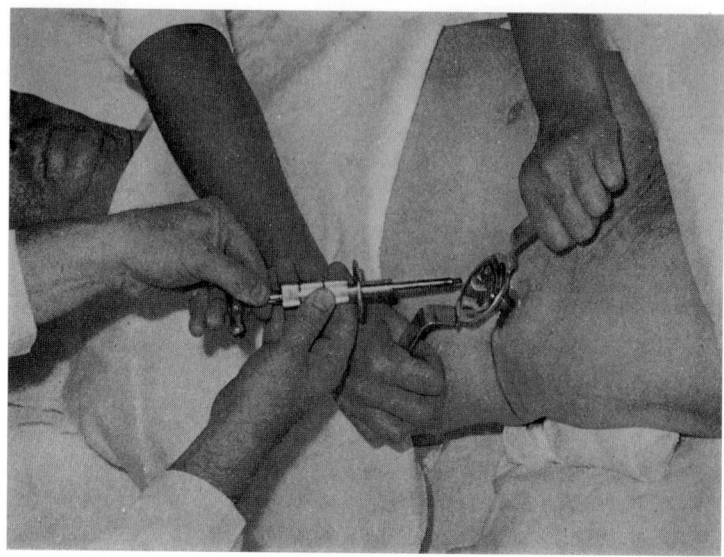

FIGURE 39c. Removal of the biopsy sample by the ejector pin. (Reproduced from *Bone Marrow and Bone Tissue: Color Atlas of Clinical Histopathology* by Rolf Burkhardt (1971), Springer-Verlag, New York, Heidelberg, Berlin.)

Manually operated boring trephine

Trephines such as Bordier's (Figure 40) are generally used for transiliac (or horizontal) biopsies (Figure 38). This approach is slightly more invasive than one through the iliac crest (vertical approach) and usually takes a little longer time (30 to 60 minitues). During this lateral approach the patient assumes a supine lateral position with semiflexion at both hip and knee. A triangular area which is known as "Bordier's Triangle" is outlined with the anterior superior iliac spine as a guide. Roughly, it is a 5 cm isolateral inverted triangle (Figure 41), the base of which is formed by the border of the iliac crest. Following preparation of the skin, and local anaesthesia [more local anaesthetic (15 to 30 ml) is needed because of the bulk of subcutaneous tissue and muscle in this region] a 2–3 cm long incision is made along the dotted line indicated in Figure 41 exposing the glistening fascia lata. The fascia itself is then incised along the direction of its fibres and the dissection is continued until the scalpel touches the subadjacent periosteum and bone. The periosteum is scraped after further local anaesthesia which helps in minimizing the discomfort. With the index finger, the surface of the bone is freed of its muscle attachments, and the plane of the body of the ilium is ascertained. The trephine is introduced and the outer sieve is fixed on the bone perpendicular to its plane (Figure 42). The procedure is then completed with the inner drilling trephine by clockwise and counterclockwise rotary motion while applying steady but gentle pressure. After the trephine has pierced the inner cortex it is rotated completely

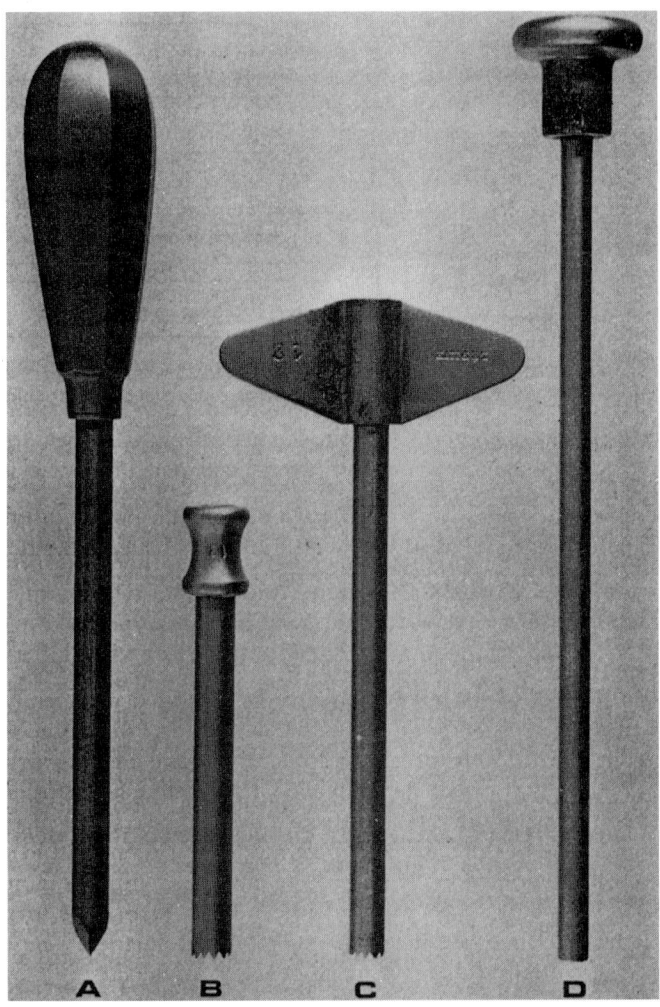

FIGURE 40. Bordier's trephine for iliac crest biopsies. (A) The trochar. (B) External cylinder with serrated edge. (C) The internal cylinder with a serrated edge. (D) The pin used to expel the biopsy from the instrument. (Reproduced from *Bone Histomorphometry: Techniques and Interpretation* by Robert R. Recker (1983), CRC Press, Inc, Boca Raton, Florida.)

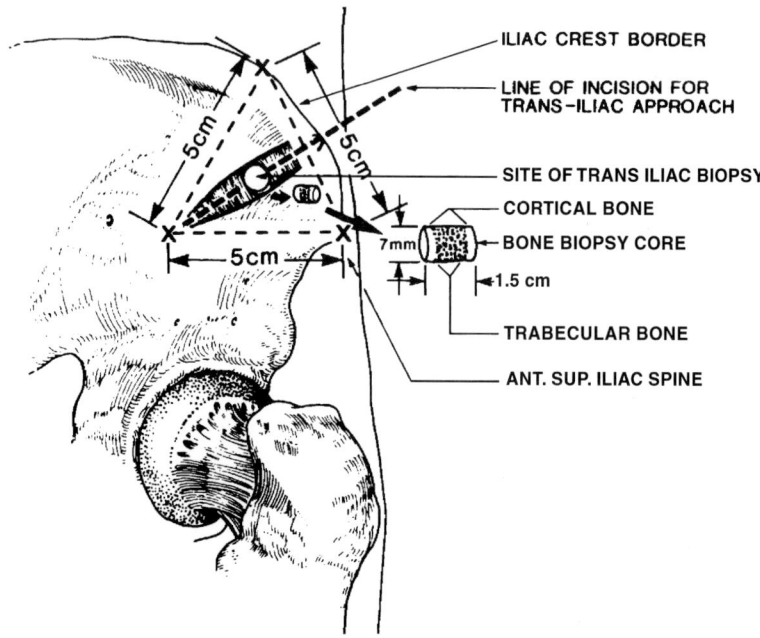

FIGURE 41. Outline of "Bordier's Triangle" and anatomic orientation for transiliac bone biopsy procedure. (Reproduced from *Bone Histomorphometry: Techniques and Interpretation* by Robert R. Recker (1983), CRC Press, Inc, Boca Raton, Florida.)

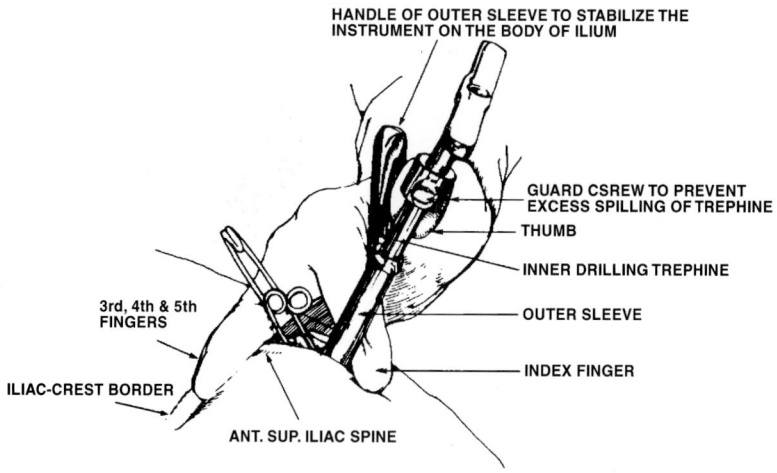

FIGURE 42. Illustrates the positioning and introduction of transiliac trephine and its components. (Reproduced from *Bone Histomorphometry: Techniques and Interpretation* by Robert R. Recker (1983), CRC Press, Inc, Boca Raton, Florida.)

2 or 3 times to achieve separation of the specimen from the inner muscle attachment. The trephine is then gently withdrawn with circular, clockwise motions and the outer sleeve is removed. Incised fascia lata is sutured with interrupted absorbable chromic material to avoid herniation of the underlying muscle. The wound is then closed in two layers using chromic suture for the subcutaneous tissue and nylon or silk for the skin. A pressure dressing is applied with elastic tape and the patient is asked to turn over and lie on the incision site for at least 15 to 20 minutes. The patient is also advised to lie on that side as much as possible for the next 24 hours although this is not an absolute necessity. Minor analgesics are usually needed for 1 or 2 days.

Although transiliac biopsy can safely be performed in 30 to 60 minutes this approach appears to be more elaborate and time consuming. There are a number of complications that are specific to a transiliac biopsy. First, a specimen may dislodge from the trephine during its withdrawal. Second, the cutting end of the trephine may separate from the shaft after penetrating the outer cortex of the ilium. In a few cases the trephine teeth may be bent or distorted as a result of undue pressure applied during the procedure. Third, haematomas are more common with this version than either the vertical or iliac crest approach. Fourth, transient neuropathy due to severance or entrapment of one of the cutaneous branches of the femoral nerve may cause hyperesthesia at the biopsy site. Fifth, pain and discomfort during and after the bone biopsy procedure is slightly more with transiliac than with the iliac crest approach. The transiliac biopsies (7–8 mm width with Bordier trephine) are mainly used by endocrinologists and osteologists for histomorphometric measurements of cortical and trabecular bone.

Bone marrow biopsy needle

There are several types of needles which are used for obtaining bone marrow biopsy samples from the sternum, anterior or posterior iliac crests. Turkel and Bethel described a microtrephine (Figure 43) (~2 mm bore) which is passed through a hollow introducing needle only slightly larger than a regular marrow aspiration needle. No skin incision is necessary and the instrument was initially designed for sternum. The latter has also been used for anterior iliac crest. However, the cylinders of bone and underlying marrow obtained with these needles are small, and they usually fragment while being prepared for processing and sectioning.

The Westerman-Jensen needle (modified Vim-Silverman needle) (Figure 44) was designed for obtaining bone marrow biopsies from the posterior iliac crest. With adequate training and experience such needles may provide adequate material but they yield smaller specimens than most other needles and technical failure of securing an adequate sample at any one given attempt remains a serious problem. In addition, the cutting blades are often splayed and occasionally completely destroyed during the procedure even after proper care has been taken. A major disadvantage in addition to delivering a rather small sample and failure to retain the core (by the Vim-Silverman and Westerman-Jensen needles) is that not infrequently the specimen is crushed and its architecture is distorted.

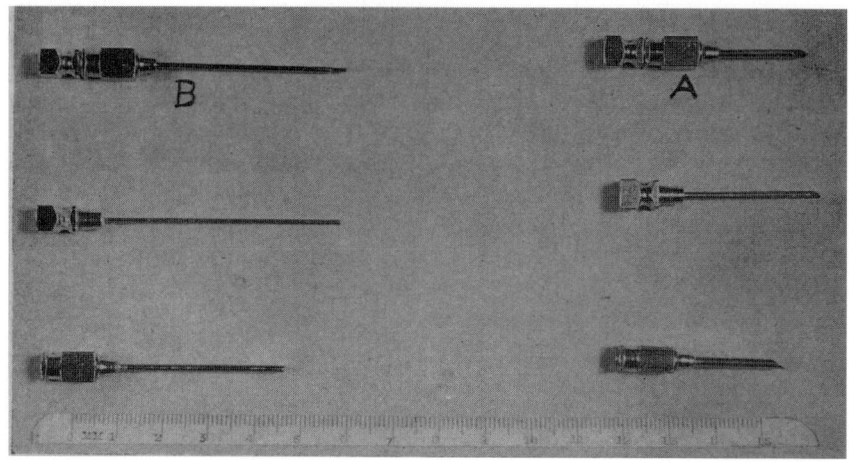

FIGURE 43. Trephine needle for bone marrow biopsy designed by Turkel and Bethel. (Reproduced from *Biopsy of bone marrow performed by a new and simple instrument* by Turkel H and Bethel, F.H.: *J. Lab. Clin. Med.*, **28**, 1246–1251, 1943)

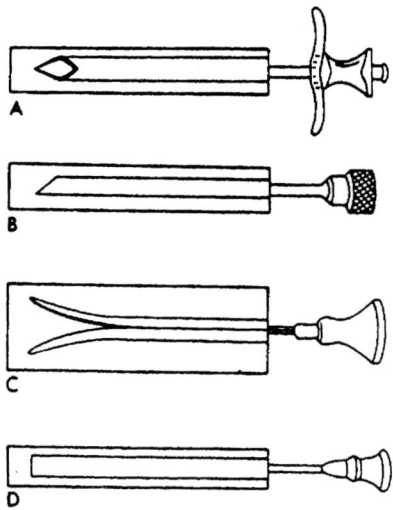

FIGURE 44. Westerman-Jensen bone marrow biopsy needle. (A)10 gauge, 4 1/4 inch long outer cannula. (B) Stylet for outer cannula. (C) Cutting prongs. (D) Stylet for cutting prongs which are used to eject bone marrow specimem. (Reproduced from *Bone Marrow Biopsy* by Perman, V. *et al.* in *Vet. Clin. N. America*, May (4), 293–309, 1974)

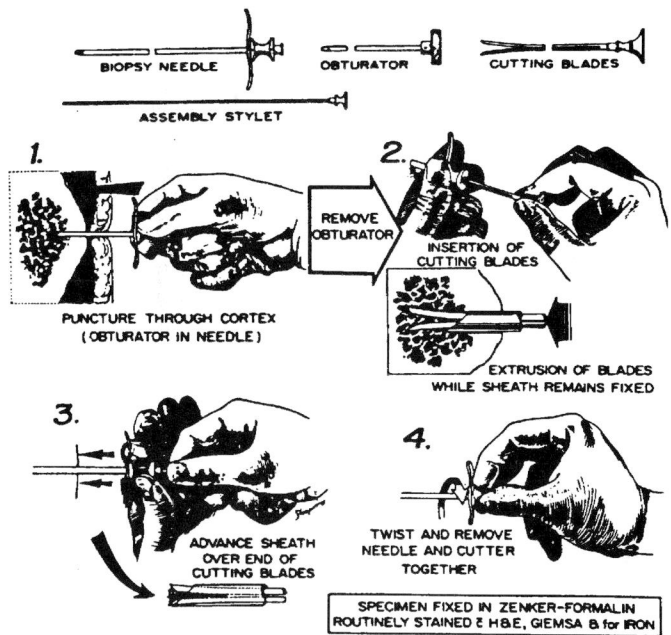

FIGURE 45. Obtaining of bone marrow biopsy from posterior iliac crest with Westerman-Jensen needle. See text for details. (Reproduced from *Needle Biopsy of Bone and Marrow* by Ellis, L.D. *et al.*, *Arch Intern Med.*, **114**, 213–221, 1964.)

Maintenance of these instruments is relatively time-consuming and requires that the cutting surface be gently rubbed with the finest possible water paper to ensure a sharp edge after every two or three usages. Any distortion of the delicate blades renders biopsy very difficult and leads to an immediate increase in crush artifact.

The biopsy technique utilizing the discussed needles in which a biopsy specimen is obtained from the posterior iliac crest is similar to that described by McFarland and Dameshek. The procedure, using the Westerman-Jensen needle, is illustrated in Figure 45. The needle has finger grips, an assembly stylet, and an obturator which locks in position in addition to being larger and sturdier than the regular Silverman needle. The patient is placed in the right or left lateral recumbent position. The needle with the obturator locked in place is inserted into the previously anaesthetised skin, subcutaneous tissue and periosteum overlying the posterior superior iliac spine. Once the cortex is penetrated and the medullary cavity reached, the stylet is unlocked and removed (Figure 45-1). The cutting blades, with the assembly stylet in place, are then inserted into the outer cannula, the assembly stylet is removed, and the blades advanced into the medullary cavity until the desired depth has been reached (Figure 45-2). The outer cannula is then advanced over the cutting blades with entrapment of the tissue (Figure 45-3), and the entire unit is then removed by a gentle twisting movement (Figure 45-4).

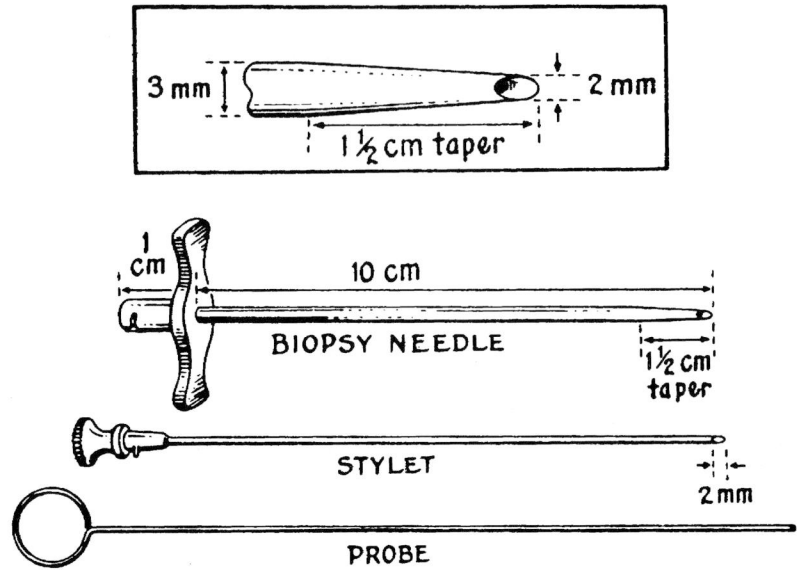

FIGURE 46. Details of the Jamshidi bone marrow biopsy needle. (Reproduced from *A New Biopsy Needle for Bone Marrow* by Jamshidi, K. *et al.*, *Scand. J. Haemat.*, **8**, 69–71, 1971.)

The specimen is removed from the cutting blades by teasing it from the tip before withdrawing the blades through the cannula. Specimens are placed immediately into an appropriate fixative, processed in a routine fashion prior to staining.

The Jamshidi needle (Figure 46) which has a tapering end appears to overcome most of the problems associated with other bone marrow biopsy needles. Sometimes, however, the sample fractures during its entry into the lumen of the needle and thus only its proximal (outer) segment (7–10 mm) is retrieved leaving the distal (inner) portion within the patient. In other cases the entire biopsy specimen remains firmly attached at its base and slips out of the needle (Figure 47) during retraction thereby requiring a second or third attempt to secure an adequate specimen. Since the Jamshidi technique requires some rocking or sculling movements with the needle to detach the biopsy specimen at its base, the needles as a result, are often bent and damaged.

These disadvantages have been overcome by incorporating a core retention device, as in the Islam bone marrow biopsy needle (Figure 48 and 49 inset). This makes it possible to cut the trabecular connections of bone very cleanly avoiding any crush artefact and also holding the core so that it does not slip out of the needle during the process of extraction (Figure 50).

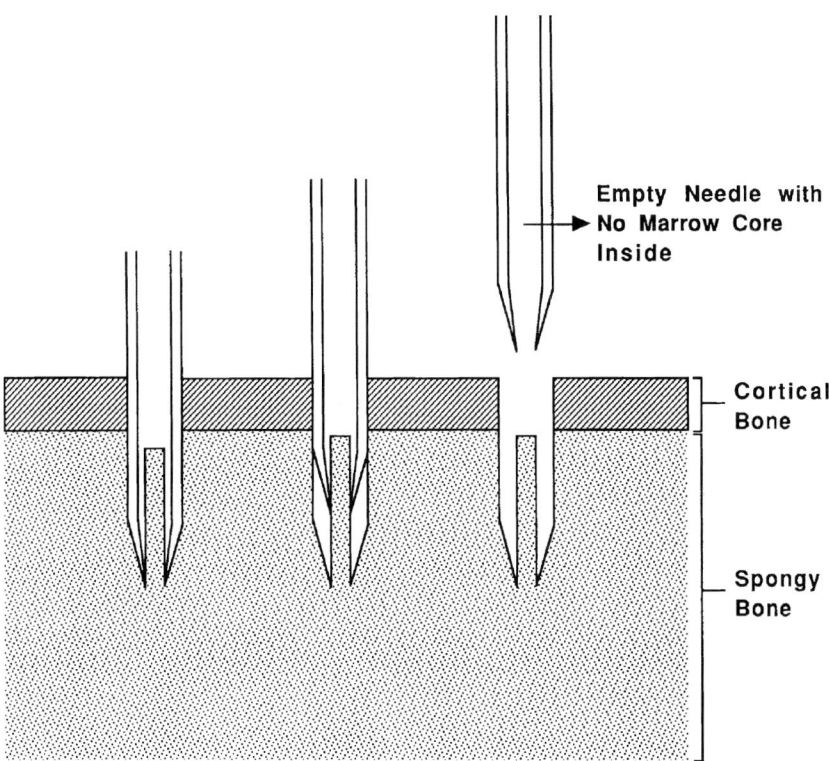

FIGURE 47. Schematic representation of the Jamshidi needle showing absence of any core securing device which may sometimes result in the loss of biopsy specimen during retraction or withdrawal of the needle.

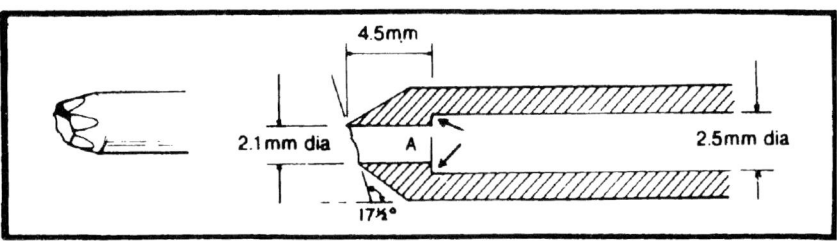

FIGURE 48. Shows details (internal view) of the distal cutting end of Islam bone marrow biopsy needle with core retention device and flueted cutting end.

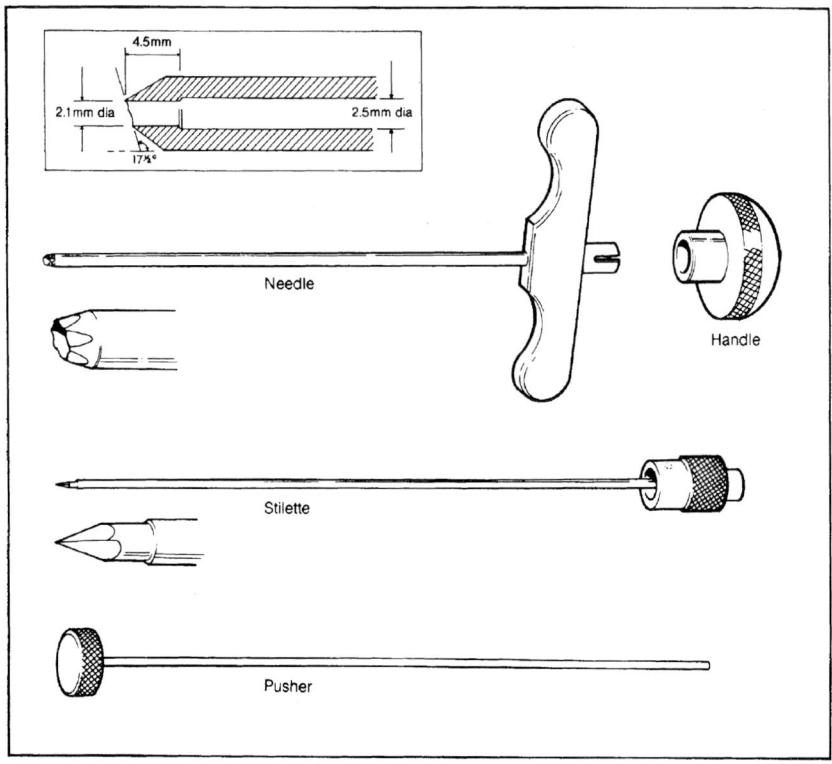

FIGURE 49. Islam bone marrow biopsy needle (see text for details).

Instrumentation

At present, the vast majority of bone marrow biopsies are obtained with either Jamshidi or Islam needles or one of the modified versions of these needles. These biopsy needles have proven to be convenient, safe, simple and easy to manipulate and without significant complications. They have now replaced almost all other methods of histologic sampling of bone and bone marrow for haematological and non-haematological diagnosis.

Both Jamshidi and Islam needles are designed to obtain bone marrow biopsies from the posterior iliac crests. In most part they offer an identical procedure except for the Islam technique where no rocking or sculling movements or change in the direction of the tip of the needle are necessary to secure the marrow core before the needle is withdrawn. With the Islam version the needle can be withdrawn with a straight pull (as it has a core retention device) without the fear of loosing the core sample.

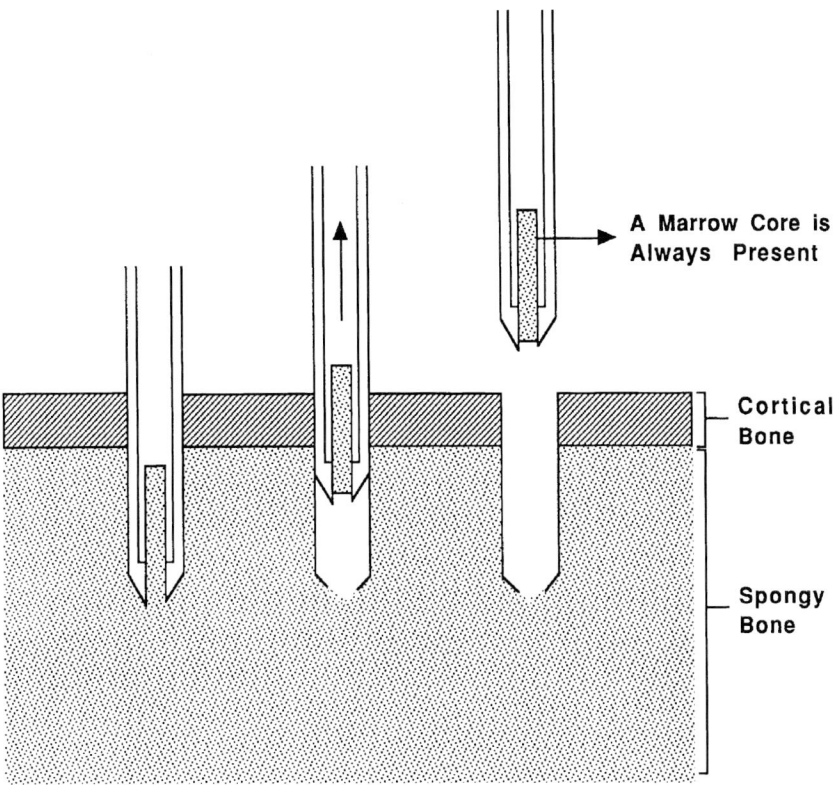

A Marrow Core is Always Present

Cortical Bone

Spongy Bone

FIGURE 50. Schematic representation of the Islam bone marrow biopsy needle illustrating the core retention device which securely holds the biopsy specimen during withdrawal of the needle.

The Islam bone marrow biopsy needle

The instrument

The steel instrument* (Figure 49) consists of four parts. *The needle* has an overall length of 122 mm, a uniform external diameter of 3.25 mm, and a constant internal diameter of 2.5 mm except for the 4.5 mm, distal portion where it is bevelled, fluted, and has a sharp cutting edge. The internal diameter of this latter segment (2.1mm) is less than the internal diameter of the longer proximal region whose interface

---

*The instrument is available in several different sizes (bore diameter and lengths). Some minor changes have recently been made to this original design.

with the distal segment ends in a short step of 0.2 mm. This specially designed distal portion cuts the trabecular connections which might keep the biopsy attached at its base and holds on to the biopsy specimen (with a lip like support) so that it does not slip out of the needle during the process of its extraction. The wider internal diameter provides ample free space within the interior of the instrument thus avoiding compression of the tissue and plugging the lumen of the needle; it also allows the specimen to be delivered freely through the proximal end of the needle. The proximal end of the instrument has been fitted with a large metal *T-bar handle* for a firm grip. In addition, it is centrally fitted with a 15 mm high round hollow metal tube to receive the stilette and also to fit the dome handle.*The stilette* is a solid shaft of 2.4 mm in diameter except for the distal portion where its diameter is 2.00 mm to fit the narrower distal cutting end. It terminates with a 3.0 mm long three-faceted sharp-pointed cutting tip which projects beyond the end of the needle in order to protect the cutting edge of the needle and to provide a means of easy penetration of the soft tissue and bony cortex. The proximal end of the stilette has a round fitting for both the domed segment and the T-bar of handle of the needle as well as a 10 mm outer shaft with serration for grip. The *pusher* (probe) is used for extrusion of the biopsy from within the needle. It is a solid shaft 1.9 mm in diameter and has an overall length of 140 mm. Its distal end is blunt and the proximal end is fitted with a 5 mm thick, flat, round knurled disc 15 mm in diameter. The *domed* segment of the T-bar handle is a semicircular smooth, solid plastic, 30 mm in diameter, 15 mm deep and has a 5 mm lightly milled edge. It rests snugly in the palm of the hand and avoids palmar pain and blister formation during the biopsy procedure. This is particularly noteworthy during the coring of a very hard bone or bone of increased density.

Schematic representation of the biopsy procedure using the Islam bone marrow biopsy needle (Figure 51)

1. The outer needle (a) with the stilette (b) in place is inserted down to the bone.
2. The cortex of the posterior ilium is then penetrated with a forward thrust and gentle rotary motion of the needle with the stilette in place. Once penetration has been achieved, the stilette is withdrawn.
3. The needle is then advanced with a slow, steady and controlled clockwise and counter-clockwise rotary motion. When an adequate depth (15–20 mm) is reached, the needle is rotated several times along its long axis and then slowly withdrawn with a straight pull. Only gentle alternating rotary motions are necessary to facilitate the withdrawal of the needle. No accessory movements (e.g. rocking or sculling) or change in the direction of the tip of the needle to break the marrow core at its base is necessary.

Schematic representation of the biopsy technique using the Islam bone marrow biopsy needle (Figure 52)

The schematic representation of the biopsy technique shows the needle wall (a), the space between the core and the internal wall of the needle (b). The free

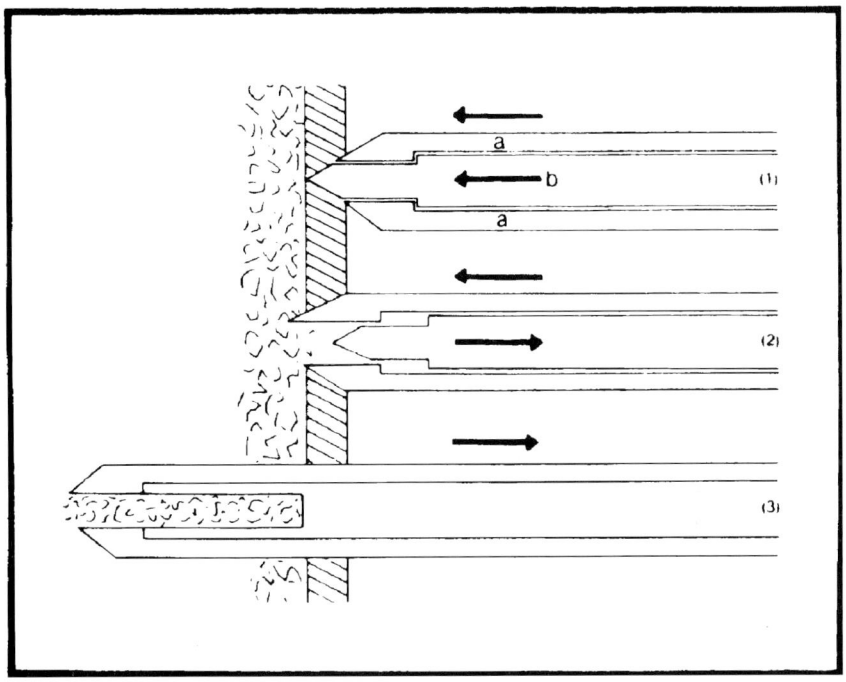

FIGURE 51. Legends incorporated in the text (see page 74).

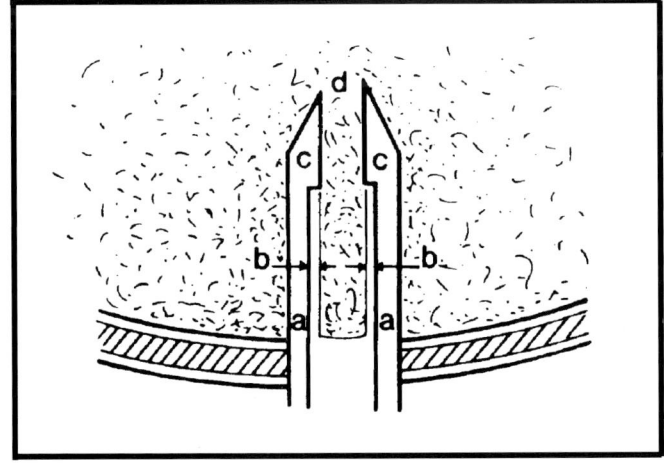

FIGURE 52. Legends incorporated in the text (see pages 74 & 76).

space between the marrow core and the internal wall of the needle helps prevent compression of the tissue and plugging the lumen of the needle. It also allows easy delivery of the core through the proximal end of the needle. The specially tooled distal cutting end (c) cuts the bony trabecular connections to the core and also assists in the retention of the core during its extraction (so that it does not slip out of the needle during its withdrawal). The base of the marrow core (d) is also shown in the illustration.

Comparison of the Islam and other (conventional) bone marrow biopsy needles

Basically, there are three types of bone marrow biopsy needles:

Figure 53 shows a representative of a class of needles which are straight hollow tubes with bevelled or serrated cutting ends. These do not have a core retention device and as a result when the marrow core is firmly attached to its base it may slip out of the tube and remain in the patient when the needle is withdrawn. Another important drawback of such needles is the fact that there is no free space between the specimen and the internal wall of the needle. As a result, a biopsy procedure with this type of needle can produce a considerable amount of crushing. Due to the absence of a free space (between the marrow core and the internal wall of the needle) the biopsy sample may also become impacted within the lumen of the needle. In such circumstances it may be difficult to push the biopsy sample out of the needle. Attempt to force the specimen out can produce a severely distorted, crushed and mangled sample as shown in Figure 53A.

Figure 54 illustrates the technique of Jamshidi needle aspiration. In the early 1970's Dr. Khosrow Jamshidi conceived the idea to provide a free space between the internal wall of the needle and the marrow core in order to avoid crushing and promoting easy delivery of the tissue through the proximal end of the needle. For some time the Jamshidi needles appeared to offer the best compromise between the straight hollow needles (Figure 53) and the much larger Bordier's trephines (Figure 40) and Burkhardt's electric myelotomy drill (Figure 37). But in a significant proportion of the cases the Jamshidi specimen becomes fractured (as shown in Figure 54A) while it is being extracted and only the smaller proximal (outer) portion (7–10 mm) is retrieved. The Jamshidi needle also does not have any core retention device and as a result sometimes when the needle is withdrawn the biopsied sample slips out of the needle and remains inside the patient thus requiring a second or third attempt to secure a biopsy sample. These repeat biopsy procedures are not without risk and are carried out at the expense of potential pain and suffering to the patient.

The Islam needle (Figures 49 and 55) was developed to incorporate the advantages of the Jamshidi version of the bone marrow biopsy needle as well as to include newly conceived features (core retention device) to negate its shortcomings. Because of the presence of core retention device the biopsied tissue is always retained within the lumen of the needle and can not slip out of the needle during the process of its extraction.

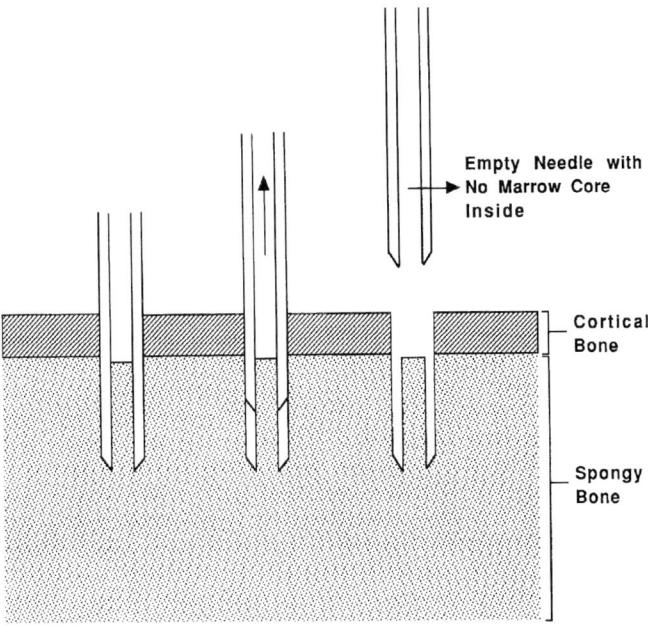

FIGURE 53. Schematic representation of the conventional bone marrow biopsy needle. Note the uniform diameter of the lumen of the needle and the absence of any free space between the marrow core and the internal wall of the needle.

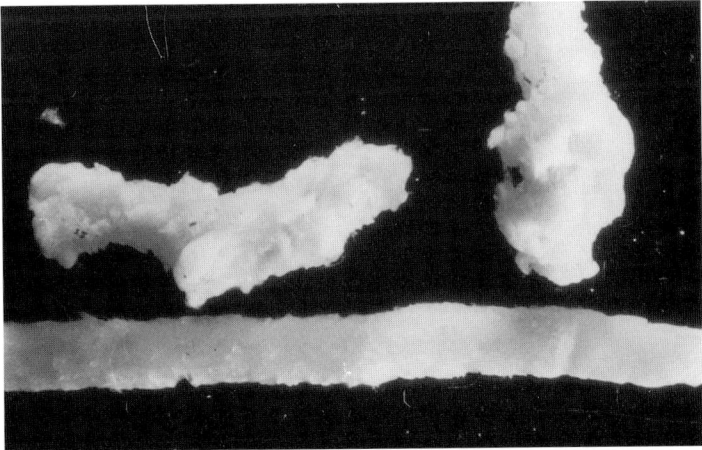

FIGURE 53A. Shows two severely crushed bone marrow biopsy samples (upper) which resulted in trying to force the impacted sample out of the needle. Lower: an undamaged biopsy sample.

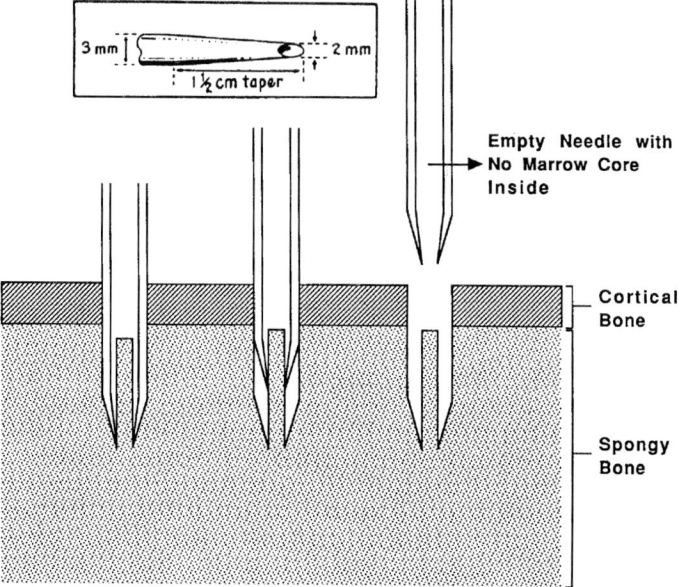

FIGURE 54. Schematic representation of the Jamshidi needle technique. Note the presence of free space between the marrow core and the internal wall of the needle. The inset illustrates the narrower distal and wider proximal end of this needle.

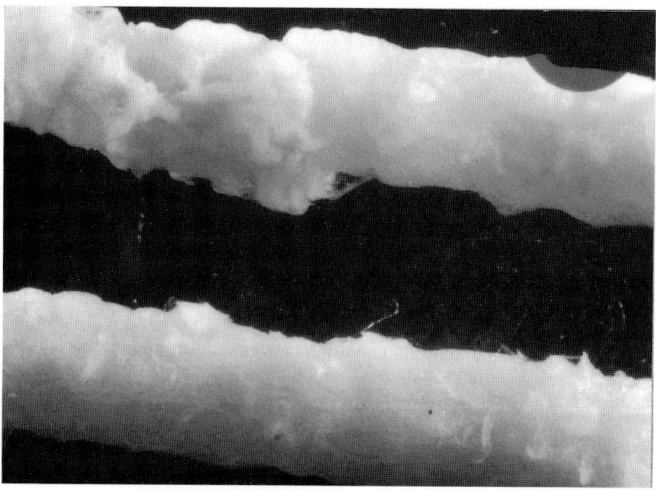

FIGURE 54A. Upper: Illustration of fractured Jamshidi derived specimen. Lower: An intact, undamaged biopsy sample.

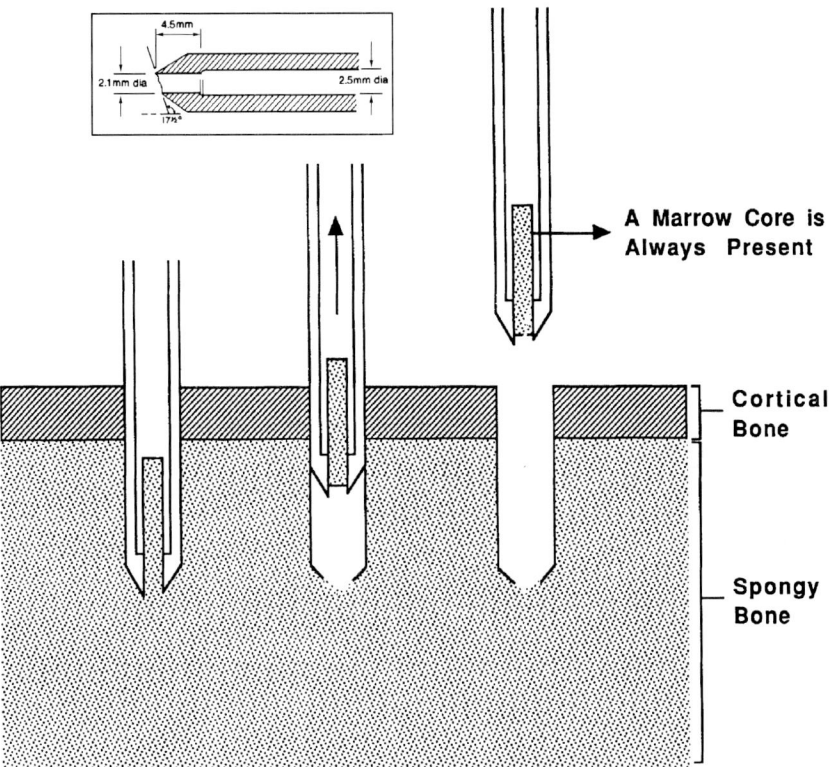

FIGURE 55. Schematic representation of the Islam needle technique. Note the presence of free space between the marrow core and the internal wall of the needle and the core retention device. The inset illustrates the core retention device in greater detail.

Biopsy Procedure

1. Site of the puncture — In adult the bone marrow biopsy is usually performed on the right or left posterior iliac crests. They form the lateral points (arrows) of the rhomboid of Michaelis and can be easily located.

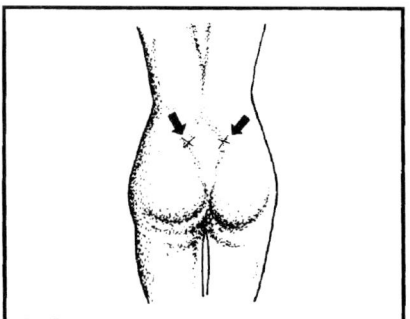

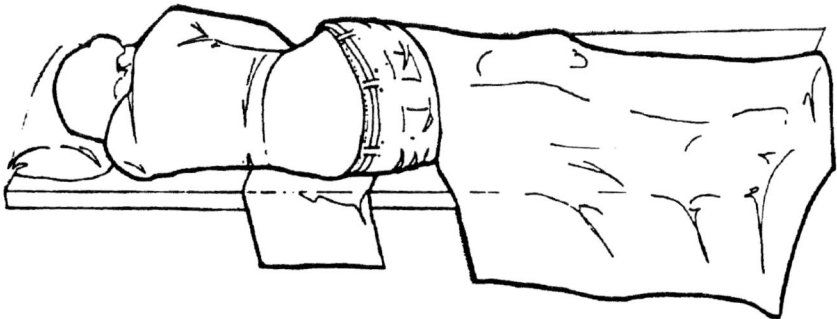

2. Position of the patient — place the patient in a right or left lateral decubitus position with the knee tops drawn up and back comfortably flexed or in a prone position with a pillow beneath the hips.

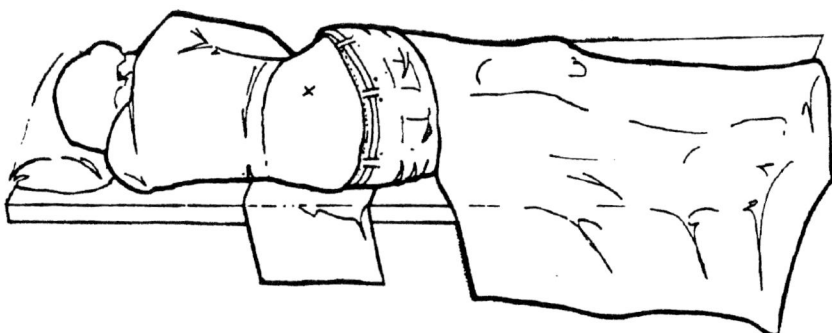

3. Once the area of the posterior iliac crest (the one selected for obtaining a bone marrow biopsy sample) is located by palpation, mark the area with thumbnail pressure and prepare the region with alcohol and iodine, and then drape.

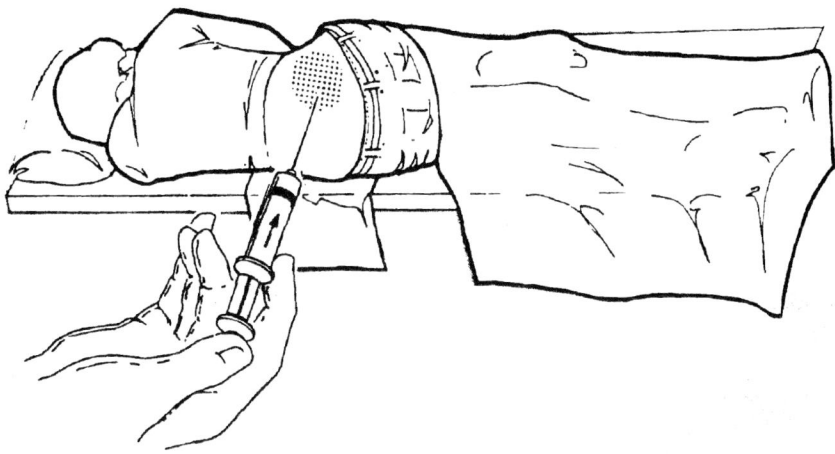

4. Infiltrate the skin, subcutaneous tissue and periosteum with a local anaesthetic (using a 25 gauge 5/8 inch needle for skin and 21 gauge 1 1/2 inch needle for soft tissue, muscle and periosteum). **Provide ample time for anaesthetic to take effect.**

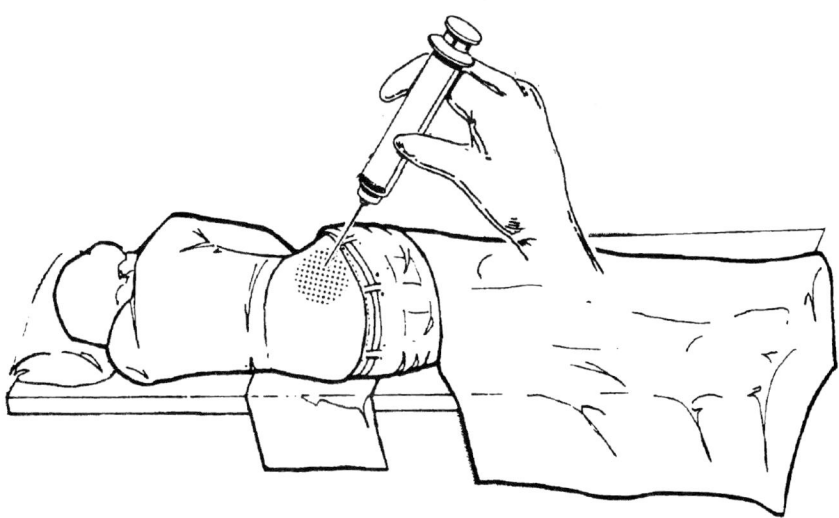

5. It is useful to probe the site with a 21 gauge 1 1/2 inch needle to see if the area is adequately anaesthetised and roughly to outline the borders of posterior iliac crest. This also gives an indication as to the depth at which the bone will be struck and desired angulation of the needle.

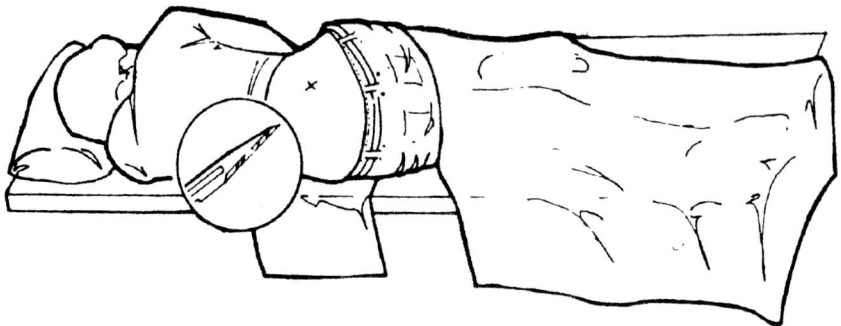

6. Make a small (3 mm) skin incision with a pointed scalpel blade over the marked area.

7. Holding of the biopsy needle — Hold the needle assembly with its domed handle rested in the palm, middle and third finger over the transverse handle, and the index finger against the shaft of the needle. The application of the index finger over the shaft (arrow) helps stabilize the needle and permits proper control.

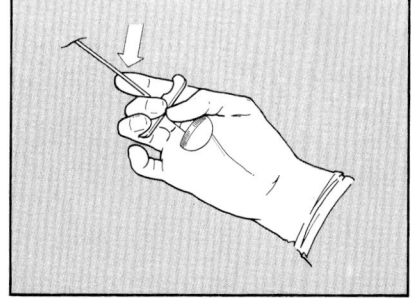

8. With the stilette and handle in place — introduce the needle through the incision and slowly advance it pointing towards the anterior superior iliac spine.

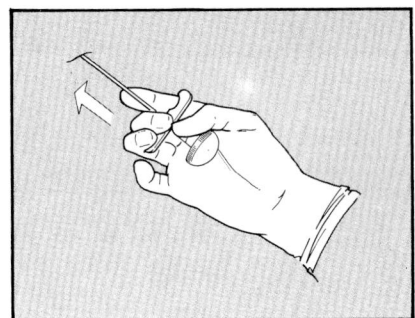

9. It is useful to put one hand over the anterior iliac crest with the middle or index finger on the anterior superior iliac spine as shown in the illustration. This approach not only helps stabilize the pelvis and patient in general but also help in the guidance of the needle towards the anterior superior iliac spine.

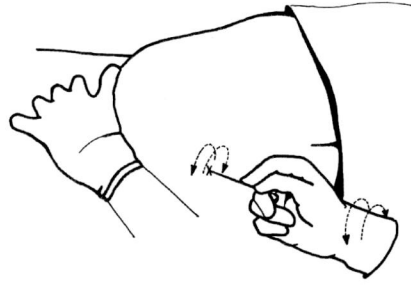

10. When the posterior iliac crest is reached, it is then penetrated by a controlled forward thrust and gentle rotary motions of the needle. Penetration beyond the cortex with the stilette in place should be avoided, as it will reduce the length of the marrow core that will be obtained.

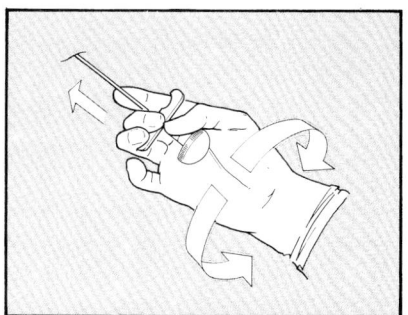

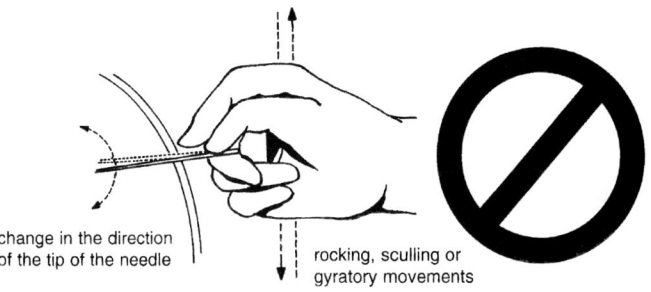

change in the direction of the tip of the needle

rocking, sculling or gyratory movements

11. While using the Islam bone marrow biopsy needle **no lateral force should be applied** during the procedure and no gyratory, rocking or sculling movements or change in the direction of the tip of the needle (as shown in the illustration) is necessary to secure the marrow core. This practice (which is essential for the Jamshidi technique) is not only unnecessary (as the Islam needle has an in built core retention device) but may also damage the needle.

12. Once the cortex is penetrated, the needle becomes locked in the cortical bone. The needle is then held in this position with the left hand (as shown in the illustration) while the right hand is used to withdraw the stilette and domed handle.

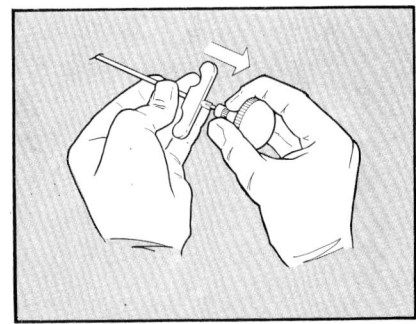

13. Remove the stilette from the domed handle and place it on the tray.

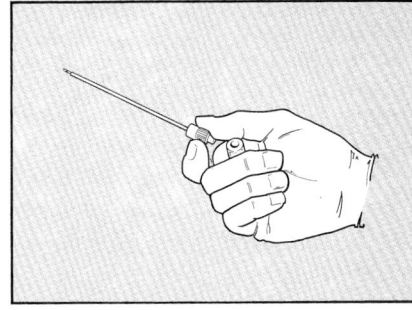

14. Replace the domed handle on the needle mount.

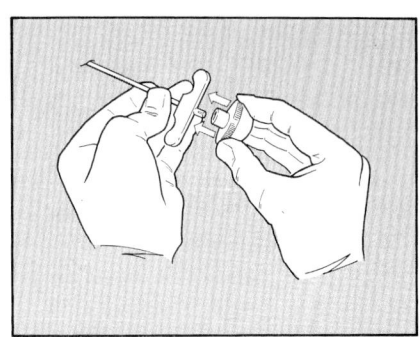

15. Advance the needle gently with slow, steady and controlled clock-wise and counter-clockwise rotary motions until an adequate depth is reached. **No lateral force** should be applied to the needle during this procedure. Failure to observe this could result in damage to the needle or injury to the patient.

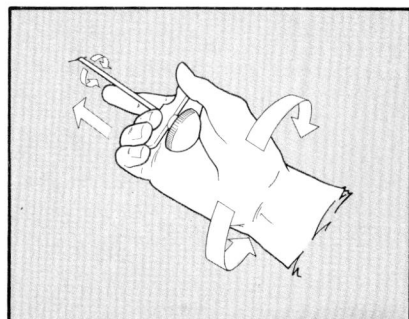

16. Rotate the needle completely (clockwise or counter-clockwise) for several times along its long axis to sever all the trabecular connections at the base of the marrow core.

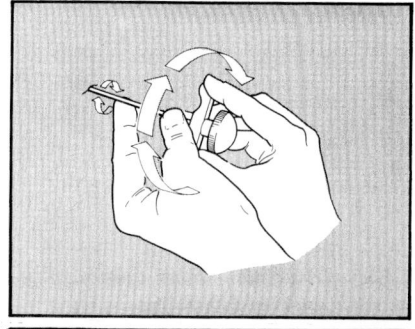

17. Withdraw the needle with a straight pull without the fear of losing the core sample. Because of the core retention device the Islam needle always holds the core captive during withdrawal of the needle. Only gentle alternating rotary motion is neces-sary to facilitate the withdrawal of the needle. Unlike the Jamshidi and other needle techniques the Islam needle procedure does not require any accessory (rocking, sculling etc.) movements or change in the direc-tion of the tip of the needle to break the marrow core at its base.

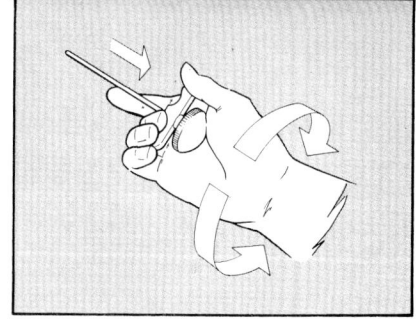

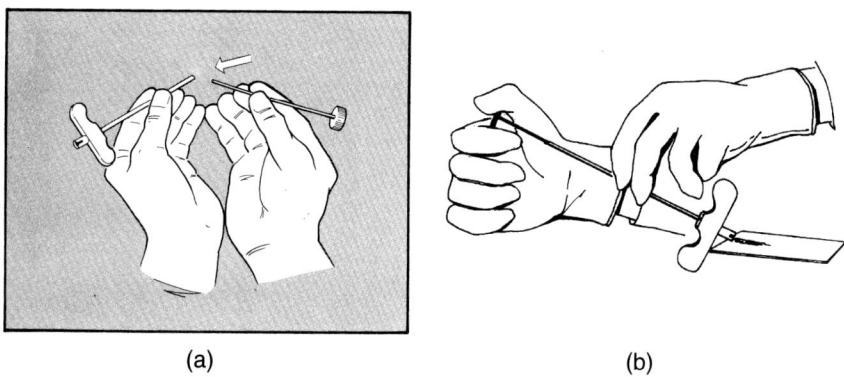

(a)   (b)

18. Once the needle is withdrawn the biopsy specimen is removed with a blunt probe which must be introduced through the distal cutting end of the needle. During the removal of the specimen, hold the needle and the probe near their tips as illustrated (a). This stabilizes the needle and the probe, prevents damage to the cutting end of the needle and helps easy delivery of the marrow core through the proximal end of the needle (b).

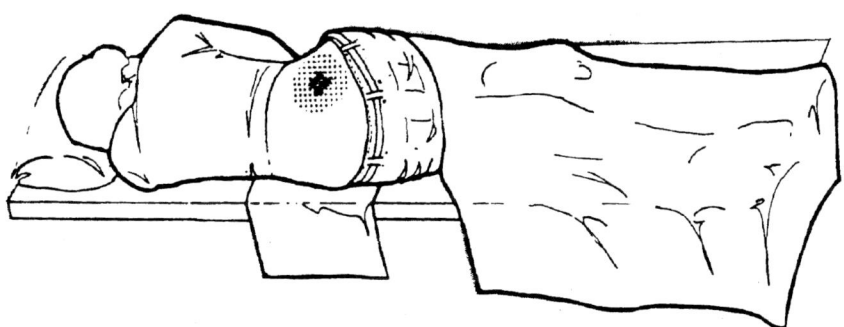

19. After the biopsy procedure, press the edges of the wound together with an adhesive tape. Apply a gauze dressing on the top of the adhessive tape and instruct the patient to lie on his/her back for 10 to 15 minutes, or longer if the patient has a low platelet count.

TIPS FOR A SUCCESSFUL PROCEDURE

The technique of obtaining a bone marrow biopsy from posterior iliac crest is simple and straightforward, and in experienced hands its performance poses no difficulty. Even experienced clinicians, however, may sometimes find it difficult, particularly in obese patients, to locate and make contact with the posterior iliac crest in an appropriate area. The following tips may be helpful in identifying and making contact with the ilium specifically at the center of the broadened, enlarged tuborosity-like, medial (paraspinal) region of the posterior iliac crest.

1. The patient is placed in the right or left lateral decubitus position.
2. The area of and surrounding the biopsy site is sterilized and adequately draped.
3. The tip of the middle finger of the right hand is placed on the end of the coccyx, and the thumb extended as much as possible over the underlying spinous processes of the lumbar vertebrae (photograph 8a). A close up view of another draped patient (photograph 8b) illustrates the position of the thumb and middle finger. The dotted line indicates the lumbar spinous processes.
4. The thumb is kept in place while the hand is rotated anti-clockwise until the tip of the index finger lies vertically in the same plane and superior to the thumb (demonstrated by dotted line) (photograph 9a and 9b). The "X" indicates the site of entry of the needle midway between the thumb and tip of the index finger.
5. The small area of the patient's lower back located in the center of the space between the thumb and index finger, is marked. (photograph 9a and 9b). This marked area lies superficial and dorsal to the target area of the posterior iliac crest. A needle introduced through the skin and into the subcutaneous tissue at this point (photograph 10) in a horizontal plane and directed towards the anterior, superior iliac spine (identified by the tip of the middle finger of the left hand, photograph 10) will hit the desired region of the medial segment of the posterior iliac crest. The aspiration biopsy and coring procedure is conducted at this locus.
6. While performing the biopsy an attempt should be made to hold the tissue mass surrounding the anterior ilium with the left hand to stabilize the patient (photograph 11) and to retain the correct orientation of the needle. The middle finger of the left hand should rest on the anterior superior iliac spine to serve as a fixed reference point and an indicator of the desired direction of the biopsy needle (see photographs 10 and 11).

The above suggestions are given to provide a guideline to help obtain adequate bone marrow biopsy samples from the posterior iliac crest. Optimally, the technique should be practiced on cadavers to perfect the procedure and to become acquainted with various adjustments that are required to accommodate factors such as the stature of the patient and size of the operator's hand.

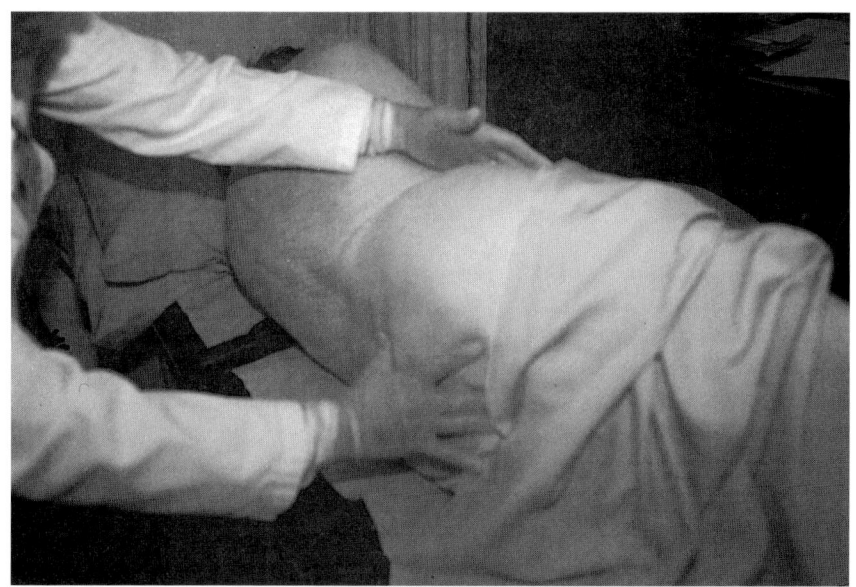

PHOTOGRAPH 8a

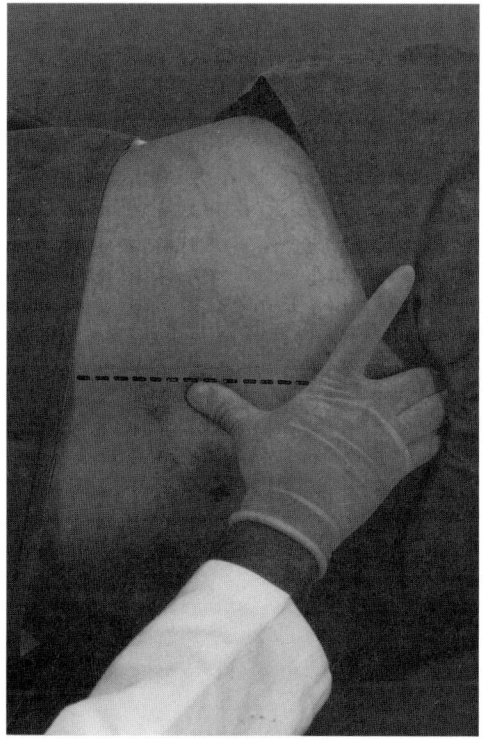

PHOTOGRAPH 8b

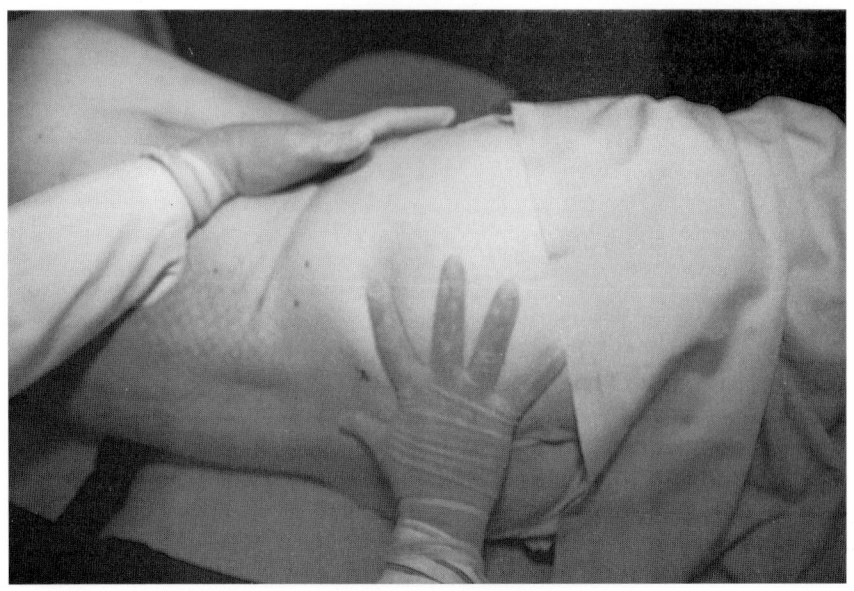

PHOTOGRAPH 9a

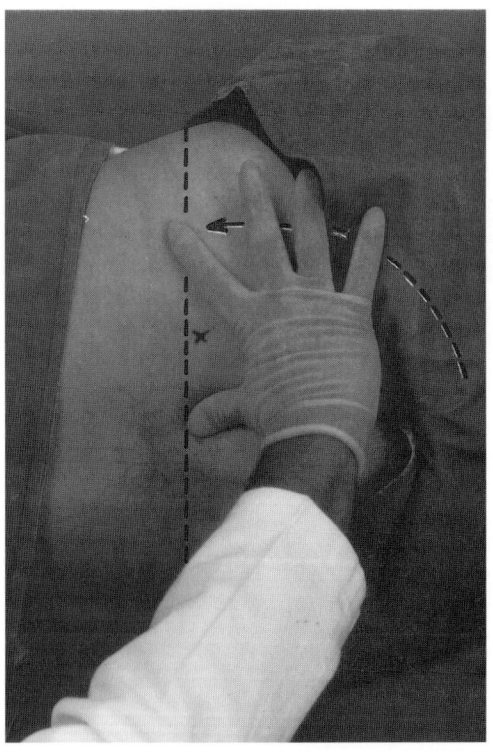

PHOTOGRAPH 9b

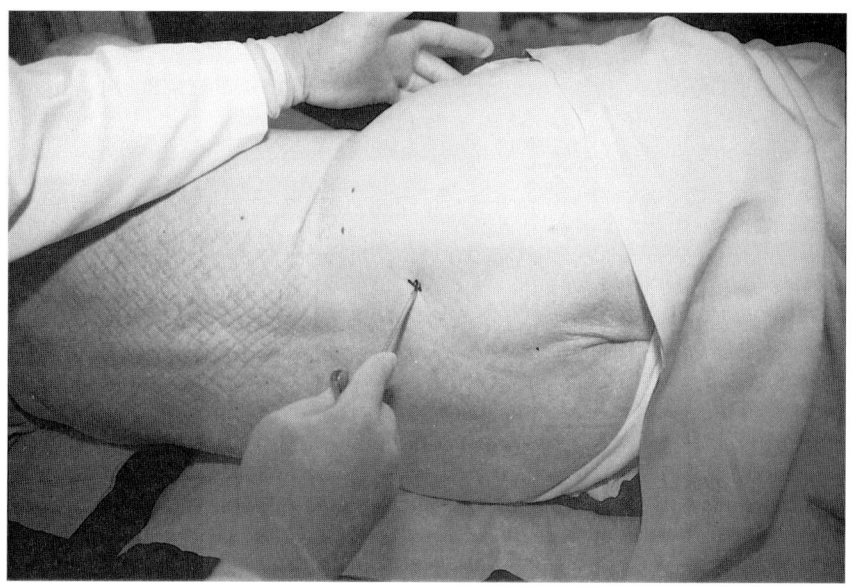

PHOTOGRAPH 10

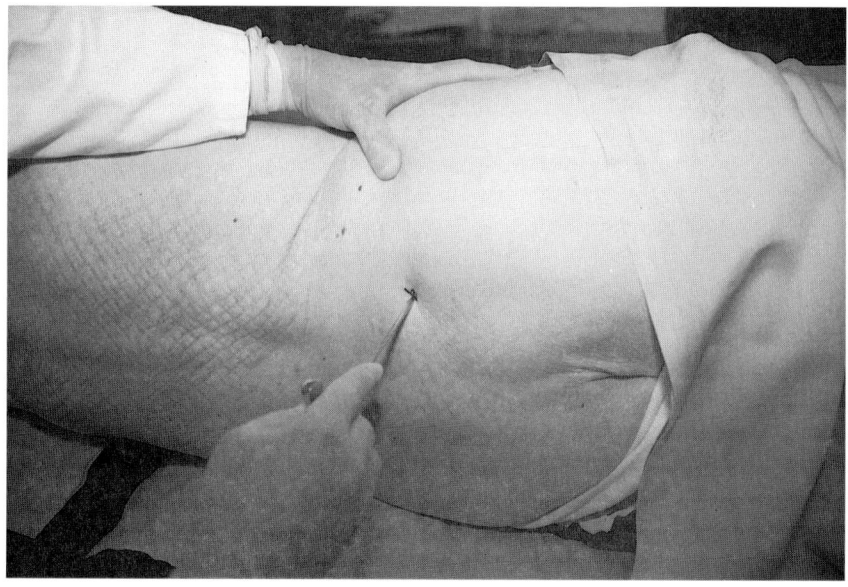

PHOTOGRAPH 11

PRECAUTION

The needle has been specially designed to obtain bone marrow biopsies from the posterior iliac crest. An important feature of the Islam bone marrow biopsy needle is the fact that it has a core retention device which makes it possible to cut and secure the core while the needle is withdrawn with a straight pull. The gyratory movements (such as rocking or sculling) or change in the direction of the tip of the needle which are necessary while using the Jamshidi or other types of needles to secure the core are not at all necessary with the Islam needles and in fact, are contraindicated as such movements will certainly damage the needle.

Although the technique of bone marrow biopsy is safe, simple and well tolerated by most patients, care must be taken while performing this procedure, particularly in obese patients. In these cases accurate localisation of the posterior iliac crest may be difficult and trauma to the sciatic nerve could ensue.

SIZE AND QUALITY OF SPECIMENS

The object of a bone marrow biopsy is to obtain a segment of bone along with an undisturbed sample of the haematopoietic cells in its medullary cavity. A long as opposed to a short bone marrow biopsy is preferred in that it may provide sufficient material for diagnosis when a smaller and perhaps less representative biopsy could be inconclusive. In adults, an adequate length and diameter of a marrow core is about 20–25 mm × 1.5–2.5 mm (Figure 34). Although an accurate diagnosis can be made from smaller biopsies when the marrow is uniformly affected, longer and larger biopsies are more useful if the lesion is more deeply placed (as detailed in the comment below and illustrated in Figures 56 and 57). Such longer and larger biopsies also provide a larger volume of tissue and a greater surface area for viewing (which may help in locating and identifying small focal lesions). The value of bilateral bone marrow biopsies in the diagnosis and management of Hodgkin's disease and non-Hodgkins lymphoma has been well established. Under ideal conditions two or three sections from each block should be reviewed. This eliminates the necessity of making diagnoses from one single view. For optimal diagnostic potential, sections derived from different depths within the same block should be evaluated.

ASPIRATION PRIOR VERSUS POST TREPHINE BIOPSY

In a marrow biopsy, an attempt should be made to obtain as much undistorted tissue as possible. Aspiration prior to coring at the same site (as practiced by some) produces considerable distortion of the marrow and therefore should be avoided. In addition aspiration prior to coring also leaves the barrel of the needle filled with marrow and blood and results in spillage during coring and removal of

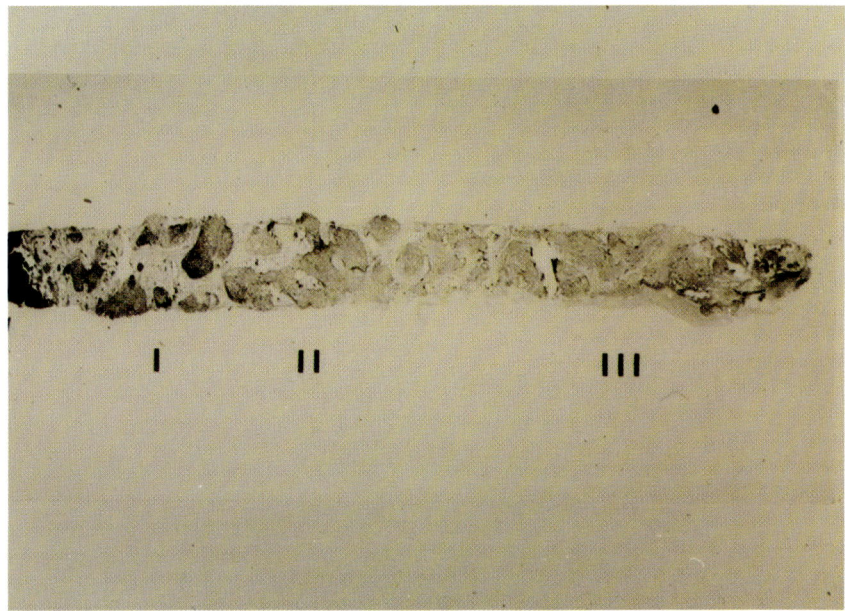

FIGURE 56. A bone marrow section of a marrow core obtained from a patient with acute lymphoblastic leukaemia in relapse, demonstrating morphological discordance in three different areas of the same section.

the biopsy from the needle. Normally bone marrow biopsy from the posterior iliac crest should be carried out first and aspiration attempted later. However, obtaining a biopsy before aspiration may cause the aspirated material to clot extra quickly due to generation of thrombin by the previous bone marrow biopsy procedure. Should an aspiration be performed first, the same puncture wound may be used for a core biopsy, but slightly different area of posterior iliac crest should be chosen for the latter. Preferably, to avoid all of the problems associated with combined aspiration and core biopsies performed at one locus, aspiration should be carried out from the sternum and a trephine biopsy from the posterior iliac crest immediately afterwards.

It is an acceptable and useful practice to use the bone marrow biopsy specimens for making imprints if proper care is taken to avoid damage to the biopsied specimen. Although the cytological preparations derived from imprints are not as cellular or as well presented as smears from aspirated samples they may prove to be confirmatory or even diagnostic when a bone marrow aspirate is unsatisfactory or yields a dry tap.

When collecting a bone marrow biopsy sample it is also important to obtain a long core biopsy as emphasized above. Biopsies of maximal length are useful particularly when the bone marrow lesion is deeply placed. This was demonstrated,

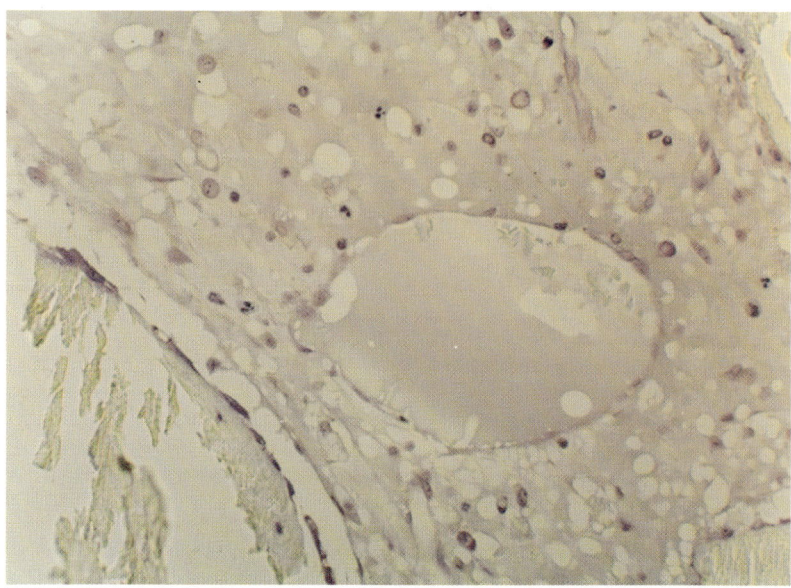

FIGURE 57a. A field from the outer portion of the marrow core (figure 56, area I) showing extremely hypocellular and grossly edematous marrow with a widely dilated sinuse and no haemopoietic activity (MMA, MGG stain).

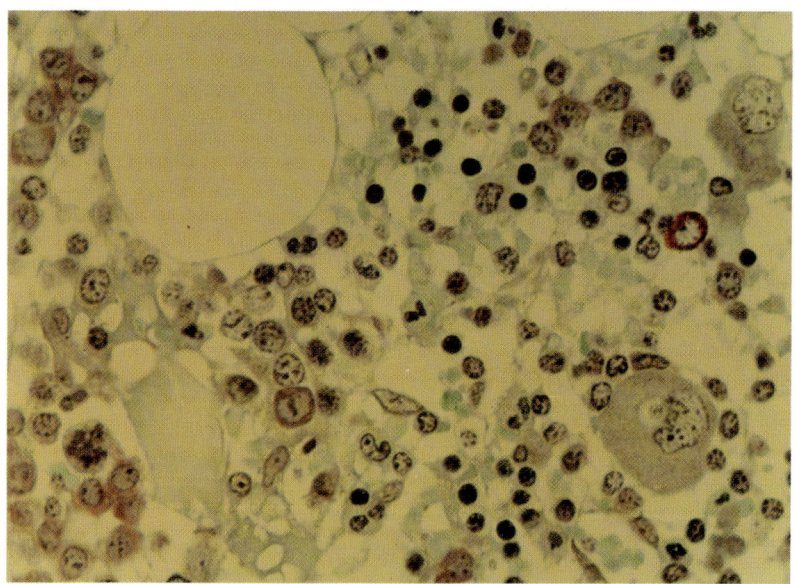

FIGURE 57b. A field from the mid portion of the marrow core (figure 56, area II) showing normal haemopoietic marrow. Note the erythropoietic and granulopoietic cells as well as the scattered megakaryocytes (MMA, MGG stain).

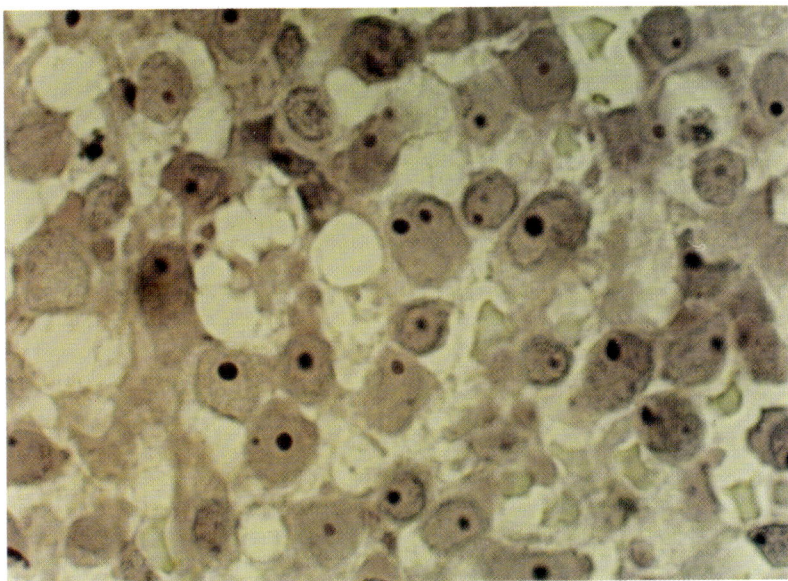

FIGURE 57c. A field from the inner portion of the marrow core (figure 56, area III) showing dense infiltration of the marrow by blast cells (MMA, MGG stain).

for example, in a case of acute lymphoblastic leukaemia which showed clinical evidence of relapse while a bone marrow aspirate sample from one site was normal and aspiration from another locus yielded an unsatisfactory specimen. Two weeks later a long core biopsy confirmed the clinical diagnosis of relapse. The histological appearance of this biopsy specimen was different in three different areas of the same section (Figure 56). The outer portion of the marrow, that is, the marrow near to the cortical bone (Figure 56 area I), showed extremely hypocellular and grossly oedematous marrow with widely dilated sinuses and no evidence of relapse (Figure 57a). The middle portion of the core (Figure 56 area II) showed normal marrow with good erythroid, granuloid and megakaryocytic activity (Figure 57b). Conversely the innermost marrow (deepest and furthest from the cortical bone) (Figure 56 area III), showed dense infiltration by blast cells (Figure 57c).

PROCESSING OF SPECIMENS

The standard preparation of sections of bone marrow biopsy specimens requires decalcification and paraffin embedding. Decalcification renders the study of the mineral phase impossible while the process of paraffin embedding distorts the marrow architecture and yields poor cytological detail. Also, paraffin-infiltrated specimens are unsuitable for the thin sectioning (less than 2 μm) that is required for detailed and precise histological analysis of a specialized multicellular tissue such as bone marrow.

Plastic embedding of undecalcified bone marrow biopsy specimens provides excellent preservation of bone marrow architecture and cellular detail. The use of a special microtome (Autocut by Reichert Jung, Germany) makes thin sectioning of mineralized bone possible. The result is improved microscopic resolution and enhanced cytology facilitating the identification of hemopoietic cells, the interpretation of cellular patterns and the formulation of diagnoses.

In recent years, various investigators have advocated plastic embedding for processing bone marrow biopsies because of the advantages this technique offers over softer embedding media such as paraffin. Various types of resins and plastics are now available for embedding bone marrow biopsies. The most commonly used ones are methyl and glycol-methacrylate. Methyl-methacrylate (MMA) is the superior embedding material, however, it has not proved successful for enzymatic and immunohistochemical applications. The water-miscible glycol-methacrylate (GMA) embedding provides good morphological detail and also yields excellent enzymatic and immuno-histochemical results. Technically it also has good stretching and mounting properties.

Some specific points in regard to the processing of bone marrow biopsies for plastic embedding and subsequent staining should be noted. An ideal fixative for morphology as well as enzyme and antigen preservation is Bouin's fixative at 4°C for 1–4 hours. For morphologic detail May-Grunwald-Giemsa stain yields the best results and also has the advantage of presenting the same staining characteristics as those obtained in similarly stained bone marrow dry film smears. It is important to note that improper tissue preparation not only augments the possibility of missing the correct diagnosis but also fosters the possibility of making erroneous interpretations.

EXAMINATION OF BIOPSY SECTIONS

A bone marrow biopsy which is of adequate size (at least 1.5–2 mm in diameter and 15 to 20 mm long), satisfactorily fixed in an appropriate fixative (like Bouin's), embedded in a suitable embedding medium (like glycol-methacrylate), sectioned at 2 μm and stained with Romanowsky's stain (e.g. May-Grunwald-Giemsa) is essential for the correct interpretation of the specimen.

An inadequacy in any of the steps mentioned above may render the specimen equivocal or unsatisfactory. This should not imply that the conventional technique of processing bone marrow biopsies in paraffin and their subsequent staining with haematoxylin and eosin makes them unsuitable for study. But there is overwhelming evidence that plastic embedded bone marrow biopsy sections offer better cytomorphological and structural detail of the marrow thereby facilitating a more accurate identification of haematopoietic cells and the formulation of the diagnosis.

In order to effectively analyze a sectioned bone marrow biopsy specimen two or more sections from different depths should be examined. The initial reading should always begin with an overall assessment of the marrow section with an examination under low power (10× objective). This insures that large cells as megakaryocytes, osteoclasts, clusters or aggregates of metastatic cells or immature haemopoietic precursor cells, macrophages, erythroblastic islets, small lymphoid nodules or lymphoid aggregates will not be missed or overlooked because of an inadequate survey. In most cases an accurate diagnosis can be made with the high dry (40×) objective. When possible (in fact this should be routinely done as the technology is now available) the sections should be stained for enzymatic and immunological markers in order to obtain the maximum possible information from a given section. The oil immersion magnification (100 x objective) is not used routinely for the examination of sections from each cases. It is required only for the study of certain nuclear or cytoplasmic details.

Although it is recognized that the cytomorphological details of haemopoietic cells in sections are not as sharply delineated as they are in Romanowsky stained smears of aspirated marrow, their presentation is certainly much better in May-Grunwald-Giemsa stained plastic embedded bone marrow biopsy sections than they are in decalcified, paraffin embedded and H & E stained preparations.

Bone marrow biopsies, particularly those from patients with haematological disorders should never be examined in the absence of available clinical information. Smears of peripheral blood and a bone marrow aspirate taken at the same time should always be examined in sequence, first the blood film and then the marrow smears. A study of the marrow biopsy sections is then undertaken. A full blood count, patients history, and laboratory findings should also be at hand prior to the morphologic analysis of the marrow.

REPORTING AND INTERPRETATION OF BIOPSY SPECIMENS

The microscopic analysis of a sectioned bone marrow biopsy should begin with careful and systematic assessment of the structural organisation of the marrow. It initiates with the study of the bony trabeculae and their lining endosteal cells, osteoblastic and osteoclastic activity. The presence of any extravasated red cells, interstitial edema, and the number and size of sinuses should also be noted as they will affect the actual estimation of overall marrow cellularity.

The intertrabecular marrow spaces which contain the haemopoietic marrow and fat cells are examined next. In thin (plastic) sections fat cells usually appear as uniform, empty, unstained spheres. Occasionally, depending on the plane of section through a fat cell, the nucleus will be seen located in an eccentric position in its complete (or incomplete) mass of cytoplasm. The vascular structures (arteries, arterioles, capillaries and sinusoids) which are seen in between and about the fat cells, haemopoietic tissue and bony trabeculae should also be closely scrutinized. Arterioles are seen infrequently and their transition to the sinusoidal system is rarely encountered. The sinusoids are lined by a single layer of endothelial cells and vary considerably in size and shape. Mature erythrocytes are found almost exclusively in the sinusoids accompanied only by occasional normoblasts or granulocytes. Megakaryocytes are often seen close to marrow sinusoids.

The haemopoietic tissue consists of a great variety of developing and mature blood cells. These free cells are mainly granulocytic and erythroid precursors at different stages of maturation including a moderate number of diffusely distributed megakaryocytes. A lesser number of lymphocytes, plasma cells, macrophages, mast cells and reticular cells are also seen. In Romanowsky stained plastic embedded (thin) bone marrow biopsy sections virtually all cells can be identified almost as readily as they are in smears of aspirated material.

Blast cells are recognised by their relatively large size, agranular deep blue cytoplasm, nucleus that manifests very delicate chromatin strands and a prominent nucleolus. Their accurate assignment to the erythroid, granulocytic or megakaryocytic cell lines however, is not always easy, especially when they are seen in isolation and devoid of accompanying mature or partially mature cells.

The report of a bone marrow biopsy should include an accurate assessment of the marrow cellularity. It is most accurately derived from sectioned material and is optimally reported (in percentage) as the aggregate volumetric ratio between the fat and haematopoietic cells. Further, the marrow space occupied by other elements such as edema, extravasated red cells, the number and size of sinuses should be carefully estimated and included in the non-haematopoietic segment of the marrow. (These factors are particularly pertinent in post therapy leukaemic marrows where the bone marrow is usually extremely hypocellular, grossly edematous and replete with dilated sinuses.) As has been indicated previously, the cellularity of the marrow diminishes with age and this physiological variation has to be taken into account in the evaluation of a given patient's tissue. The next step in the evaluation of the bone marrow should address the qualitative and quantitative aspects of erythropoiesis, granulopoiesis, megakaryopoiesis and the presence or absence of any abnormal cells. Then an assesment of the marrow fibre (reticulin or collagen) content should be made. If special staining procedures (enzyme and immunohistochemistry) are ran, these preparations should be examined and the findings reported. Finally a comment should be made as to the reviewer's overall impression of the marrow.

FORMAT FOR AN EFFECTIVE AND USEFUL REPORT

1. **Site**: indicate the site(s) where the biopsy was obtained. Report for example, whether the right or left posterior iliac crest was utilized. If another site was biopsied for marrow smears this should also be noted. Should a core and aspiration biopsy be obtained at the same site the sequence of the procedures should be given. List the anaesthetic(s) used.

2. **Bony trabeculae**: an accurate assessment of the bony trabeculae will include for example, whether they are of normal thickness or thin (osteoporosis), very thick with a large seam of osteoid (osteomalacia) or very thick and irregular with some degree of marrow fibrosis (osteomyelosclerosis). An assessment should also be made at the same time of the endosteum, osteoblastic and osteoclastic activity.

3. **Edema and extravasation of red cells**: the presence of edema (as often seen in post-therapy marrows) and extravasation of erythrocytes (seen in leukaemic as well as non-malignant conditions) should be noted and recorded when present.

4. **Vascular structures**: the number and size of the venous sinuses can be important (they are enlarged and increased in number, for example in some myeloproliferative conditions and following chemotherapy). The status of the arteries, arterioles and capillaries should be noted (e.g amyloid deposits).

5. **Fat cells**: they normally comprise about 50% of the volume of haemopoietic marrow in the normal adult. Their presence in excess of or less than this value is an indicator of hypo and hyper haemopoietic activity. The absolute absence of adipose cells is a very significant event associated typically with malignant proliferations. Normally fat cells appear as uniform, unilocular spheres and usually are uniformly distributed throughout the marrow. They may also be seen in clusters (occasionally in large patches) and concentrated around some bony trabeculae.

6. **Overall cellularity**: in sections the hemopoietic cellularity can be quantified and expressed as a percentage of the volume of marrow. For example a leukaemic marrow may be packed with malignant cells with less than 10% of the volume comprised of fat cells. Cellularity may then be described as over 90%. Whereas following therapy with the removal of the leukaemic cells the marrow may become hypocellular with less than 20% cellular elements (residual leukaemia and inflammatory cells and stromal elements) while rest of the marrow may show edema, widely dilated sinuses and only a small number of developing multilocular fat cells.

7. **Erythropoiesis**: the level of activity should be indicated as normal, increased or decreased; maturation sequence (normoblastic vs megaloblastic); cytologic abnormalities such as dyserythropoietic changes, etc.

8. **Granulopoiesis**: the level of activity should be indicated as normal, increased or decreased; maturation sequence (i.e. whether all stages of maturation are represented or if there is a maturation arrest); cytologic abnormalities such as dysgranulopoiesis (giant metamyelocytes, Pelger-Huet forms etc.); the presence and localisation of the number of myeloblasts and promyelocytes.

9. **Megakaryopoiesis**: a numerical assesment should be made (increased, normal or decreased); consider the maturation sequence, platelet production, pleomorphism, cytologic abnormalities such as dysmegakaryopoiesis (small mononuclear or multinucleated forms etc.).

10. **Plasma cell series**: a numerical assessment should be made (expressed in percentage of haemopoietic cells). Consider the maturation process, inclusion bodies, abnormalities or neoplastic changes. The distribution pattern of the plasma cells is important in reactive vs malignant conditions. Note whether they are perivascular, diffuse, scattered or clustered.

11. **Lymphocyte series**: give a numerical assessment of the lymphocytes (expressed as percentage of the haemopoietic cells in the biopsy). Indicate the presence of lymphoid nodules, germinal centers, morphologic abnormalities (large, small, cleaved cells, presence of nucleoli), their distribution should be noted e.g. diffuse, interstitial, clustered, and paratrabecular.

12. **Eosinophils and basophils**: a numerical assessment should be made (expressed in percentage of haemopoietic cells). Note any morphologic abnormalities and any infiltrative pattern if present.

13. **Iron stores**: estimate the level of content (normal, increased or decreased). The histological specimen allows more accurate evaluation of iron stores than do marrow smears, isolated spicules, or sections of bone marrow clots. The estimation of haemosiderin content is more accurately made in tissue sections because they are usually larger specimens and have a more uniform thickness than the adherent marrow units in smears. Routinely, both smears and sections should be examined for iron stores. The presence or absence of ring sideroblasts though identifiable in sections are best visualized in aspirate smears.

14. **Miscellaneous**: record the presence of macrophages, mast cells, granulomas, amyloidosis, gelatinous transformation of fat, pathologic lesions of the bone, and metastatic neoplasms etc.

15. **Differential cell count**: it is not practical to perform a standard bone marrow cell differential count on a bone marrow (paraffin or plastic embedded) section. However, the identification of essentially all cells is more effectively accomplished with plastic embedded, Romanowsky stained thin sections than with paraffin embedded, H&E stained preparations. When a bone marrow cell differential count is required it is best carried out on dry film smears. See Table 1 for the ranges of the normal bone marrow differential count.

16. **Marrow fibre content**: indicate whether the fibre content is normal or increased. If increased, note whether the augmentation is due to reticulin or collagen or both.

17. **Enzyme and immunological marker Studies**: if carried out, they should be analysed and reported.

18. **Conclusion**: give an overall impression as to whether the marrow is normal or abnormal. If abnormal, identify the specific abnormality whenever possible (e.g. acute or chronic myeloid leukaemia, chronic lymphocytic leukaemia, aplastic anaemia etc). Any other studies that may be required to make a specific diagnosis should also be identified.

EXAMPLES OF DESCRIPTIONS OF SECTIONS FROM REPRESENTATIVE HAEMATOLOGIC DISEASES

Normal Healthy Bone Marrow

Bone marrow biopsy (2 mm × 20 mm) obtained from the right posterior iliac crest under local anaesthesia. Overall cellularity within normal limits. Erythropoiesis active and normoblastic. Granulopoiesis active and presents all stages of maturation. Megakaryocytes plentiful. Gomori's reticulin stain shows a normal reticulin pattern. Iron stores normal.

Comment

The marrow appearance is normal.

Acute Leukaemia

Bone marrow biopsy (2 mm × 18 mm) obtained from the right posterior iliac crest using a Jamshidi/Islam needle under local anaesthesia. Cellularity over 90% and fat less than 10%. Erythropoiesis markedly depressed, only scattered and occasional small clusters of erythroid precursors seen. Granulopoiesis markedly depressed, only a few mature forms seen. Megakaryocytes absent. There is marked infiltration of the marrow by sheets of blast cells. Gomori's reticulin stain shows no increase in reticulin or collagen fibres.

Comment

The marrow appearance is consistent with the diagnosis of **acute leukaemia**. Morphologically the blast cells are difficult to characterise either as myeloblasts or lymphoblasts. However, if enzymatic and immunostaining are carried out on the sections and if majority of the blast cells are myeloperoxidase and CD13, 33 (and ± 34) positive then the diagnosis of **acute myeloblastic leukaemia** can be made.

Post Therapy Bone Marrow

Bone marrow biopsy (2 mm × 15 mm) obtained from the left posterior iliac crest under local anaesthesia, one week following induction chemotherapy. Overall cellularity markedly reduced (cellularity 15–20%. Fat 10–15%, remainder is edema). Cells now present consist mostly of lymphocytes, plasma cells, tissue mast cells and macrophages. Few scattered and occasional clusters of (residual) blast cells seen (less than 10%). Haemopoietic activity remains depressed. There is gross edema, some extravasation of red cells and increased number of widely dilated sinuses. There is marked pericapillary infiltration of plasma cells.

Comment

Post therapy marrow which shows presence of a small number (< 10%) of residual blasts.

Chronic Myeloid Leukaemia

Bone marrow biopsy (2 mm × 22 mm) obtained from the right posterior iliac crest under local anaesthesia. Overall cellularity markedly increased (over 97%). Only few scattered remaining fat cells (less than 3%) were seen. Erythropoiesis markedly depressed, few scattered and occasional small islands of erythroid precursors (mostly at the same stage of maturation) were seen. Granulopoieis markedly increased, mostly mature (myelocytes, metamyelocytes and segmented) forms were seen. Blast cells prominent near some bony trabeculae. Occasional small clusters of blasts were also observed in the central intertrabecular marrow spaces. Megakaryocytes (clustered and scattered) increased and show dysplastic changes. Some (large) megakaryocytes were seen close to marrow sinusoids.

Comment

The marrow appearance is consistent with the diagnosis of **chronic myeloid leukaemia**. Chromosome analysis and a leukocyte alkaline phosphatase score would help validate the diagnosis.

Chronic lymphocytic Leukaemia

Bone marrow biopsy (2 mm × 20 mm) obtained from the right posterior iliac crest under local anaesthesia. Overall cellularity markedly increased (80–90%). There is a reciprocal reduction of the fat cells which now constitute about 10–20% of the marrow. There is diffuse (interstitial infiltration of varied density) and nodular infiltration of the marrow with mostly mature-appearing small lymphocytes. The infiltration is particularly dense in the perisinusoidal regions. A variable number of mast cells and plasma cells are seen. Erythropoiesis is normoblastic but its activity is reduced. Granulopoietic activity is also reduced but presents all stages of maturation. Megakaryocytes are seen but reduced in number. Gomori's reticulin stain shows a fine network of reticulin fibres present mostly in and around the lymphoid nodules and in the densely infiltrated areas. Iron stores normal.

Comment

The marrow appearance is consistent with the diagnosis of **chronic lymphocytic leukaemia**. This can be further substantiated if the lymphocytes are CD 5 and CD19/20 positive.

Aplastic Anaemia

Bone marrow biopsy (2 mm × 20 mm) obtained from the right posterior iliac crest under local anaesthesia. Overall cellularity markedly reduced (less than 10–15%). Fat cells (mostly uniform in size and unilocular) markedly increased (75–80%). There is some edema, but no extravasation of red cells and vascular system (sinusoids and capillaries) are prominent. Cells now present consist mostly of mature lymphocytes, plasma cells, tissue mast cells and macrophages. Erythropoiesis is markedly depressed, only a few small clusters of erythroid precursors, mostly at the same stage of maturation ("hot spots") are seen. Granulopoiesis markedly depressed, only a small number of mature myeloid precursors seen. Megakaryocytes absent.

Comment

The marrow appearance is consistent with the diagnosis of **severe aplastic anaemia**.

COMMON PROBLEMS AND THEIR RESOLUTION

Loss of or Failure to Obtain a Core Biopsy

Although a satisfactory sample of bone marrow can be obtained without much difficulty from the posterior iliac crest (the site most commonly used at the present time) with the use of unimproved, standard needles, occasionally a core sample may slip out of the needle during its withdrawal and remain inside the patient. This problem is often encountered with Jamshidi and somewhat similar types of needles as they do not have a biopsy specimen retention device. In such circumstances it is necessary to re-insert the needle with its stilette in place and advance the needle into the bone in a slightly different direction in order to secure another sample. Sometimes, however, especially in cases of severe myelosclerosis or osteoporosis a marrow sample remains unobtained even with repeated attempts. In such circumstances a needle with a core securing device (such as the one in the Islam bone marrow biopsy needle) may prove to be useful. In patients with osteoporosis the needle should be introduced very carefully into the bone and marrow should be cored with slow, steady, clockwise and counter-clockwise rotary motion with a gentle forward thrust. Otherwise the soft osteoporotic marrow will crumble and little or no marrow tissue, or only a small crushed sample may remain within the lumen of the needle upon its withdrawal from the patient.

INDICATIONS

The indications for bone marrow biopsies are manyfold. The information obtained from the combined study of bone marrow aspirate and bone marrow biopsies particularly in haematological disorders is markedly enhanced over that obtained when only one of the procedure is elected. Indeed, because the technique has become so convenient and practical as well as yielding tissue with excellent histologic and cytomorphologic detail that any patient undergoing a bone marrow aspiration should concomitantly have a bone marrow biopsy.

In *haematology* bone marrow biopsies are either required or yield significant information for the diagnosis and differential diagnosis of hypoplasias and aplasias; for the diagnosis, differential diagnosis, and classification of myelo- and lymphoproliferative disorders, for the documentation of ontogeny and evolution of a disease process, for monitoring therapy and detection of residual disease, to evaluate factors of possible prognostic significance, and for the assessment of haematopoietic tissue and stromal response at diagnosis, post chemotherapy and before and after autografts and transplants.

Specific indications for a core bone marrow biopsy *in haematological disorders* are all cases of acute and chronic leukaemia, hypoplasia and aplasia, myelodysplastic syndromes, cytopenias and conditions with potentially increased marrow reticulin and/or collagen. The need for biopsy in other conditions such as Hodgkin's disease, non-Hodgkin's lymphoma and multiple myeloma has already been established.

In *internal medicine* bone marrow biopsy is useful in many endocrine disorders, in disturbances of renal function, for the detection of amylodosis, in autoimmune disorders particularly for the assessment of the walls of blood vessels, for the diagnosis of granulomatous diseases and various other non-specific conditions.

Bone marrow biopsy is diagnostic in storage diseases such as Gaucher's disease and may be useful in histoplasmosis, toxoplasmosis, Q fever, giant cell arteritis, in mesenchymal and collagen disorders, and in rare metabolic disturbances such as hypophosphatasia. Bone marrow biopsy is also indicated in any condition involving alterations in the formation and resorption of bone which may occur in a wide variety diseases either primarily or secondarily, e.g. Paget's disease, osteoporosis in intestinal malabsorption, in vitamine and mineral deficiencies, in certain congenital disorders and malignancies.

In *non-haematologic malignancies* a bone marrow biopsy can provide evidence of metastases, and information useful in the evaluation of marrow function and reserve before, during and after cytotoxic therapy, and the early recognition of dysplastic changes which may herald the development of a haematologic malignancy (often as a consequence of cytotoxic therapy).

INFORMATION OBTAINABLE FROM A SAMPLE

The information that is obtainable from a bone marrow biopsy has consistently been impressive. As indicated previously, in haematological disorders in which the marrow is either hypocellular (as in cases of aplastic anaemia) or hypercellular (as in cases of leukaemia and other myelo-and lymphoproliferative disorders) a bone marrow biopsy provides critical information. In cases where there is an increase in marrow reticulin and/or collagen, the results of aspiration are usually unsatisfactory (dry tap), and a bone marrow biopsy not only becomes mandatory but is the only available vehicle which can yield a morphologic diagnosis. In sections of bone marrow biopsy specimens overall cellularity as well as quantitative and qualitative cytologic features can be accurately assessed for their diagnostic and prognostic significance.

Aplastic Anaemia

In patients clinically suspected of having aplastic anaemia, a bone marrow biopsy is essential not only to exclude other causes (such as refractory anaemia, hairy cell leukaemia, myelofibrosis, malignant lymphoma, metastatic carcinoma) that might be responsible for the clinical presentation but also establish the definitive diagnosis. In patients with aplastic anaemia a bone marrow dry film smear alone is rarely sufficiently diagnostic.

In aplastic anaemia bone marrow biopsy demonstrates a drastic reduction in haematopoietic tissue with a corresponding increase in fat cells. A small number of (residual) erythroblastic islands (aggregates of erythroid precursors which are at the same stage of maturation), so-called "hot spots", are seen located close to the marrow sinusoids and near the bony trabeculae (personal observation). These hot spots and some additional features of possible prognostic significance such as an increase in inflammatory cells (plasma cells, lymphocytes, tissue mast cells and macrophages) are more accurately visualised and quantified in a bone marrow biopsy sections than in dry film smears.

Acute and Chronic Myeloid Leukaemia

In some instances of these conditions definitive pathological features may exist that can only be identified and documented in bone marrow biopsy sections. A new classification of AML (with possible prognostic implications) has recently been proposed on the basis of observations on plastic embedded sections of solid tissue specimens. The evaluation of a bone marrow biopsy is also the most effective means of validating the presumptive induction of complete remission and monitoring the effects of therapy as compared with the examination of peripheral blood or bone marrow aspirates alone. Sectioned biopsies may also provide a means of understanding of the role of the marrow microenvironment during reconstitution of the marrow following therapy. In AML following chemotherapy, and CML after autografting, micro-anatomic relationships has been observed between the regenerating haematopoietic cells and the stromal cells (fat, fibroblast-like and endothelial cells). Haemopoietic regeneration was seen to occur preferentially within areas of structured fat (areas of tissue consisting of large uniform unilocular fat cells in close apposition) and in close vicinity of vascular endothelial cells suggesting the existence of a functional role (through the elaboration and interaction of cytokines) between the two. The biopsy sections also provide means of exploring and understanding the ontogeny and etiology of these disorders.

Chronic Lymphocytic Leukaemia

In the early stages of chronic lymphocytic leukaemia (CLL) there may be an absence of or only minimal diffuse infiltration of the marrow by small round (mature) lymphocytes, with or without the development of nodular aggregates. With progression of the disease both forms of CLL (diffuse and nodular) encroach upon the normal haematopoietic population and until it is completely replaced by the lymphoid cells. Statistical analysis of untreated patients with CLL have shown that the histologic pattern of bone marrow involvement has prognostic significance with a shorter median survival for the diffuse and a longer survival for the nodular variety.

Myelodysplastic Syndromes (MDS)

Myelodysplastic Syndromes are characterised by qualitative and quantitative defects in haematopoiesis. Abnormalities occur in all three cell lines and are observed in smears of aspirates, in bone marrow biopsy sections and by electron microscopy. There is usually a single or combined cytopenia and the bone marrow may be normo-, hypo- or hypercellular. One of the characteristic features of these conditions is the abnormal clustering of immature myeloid precursor cells popularly termed "ALIPs" (abnormal localisation of immature precursors). This particular feature of possible prognostic significance can only be seen in sections of bone marrow biopsy specimens.

Chronic Myeloproliferative Disorders (MPD)

In these conditions (e.g. polycythaemia vera (PV), chronic myeloid leukaemia (CML), idiopathic thrombocythaemia (IT), myelofibrosis (MF) and osteomyelo-sclerosis) distinctive morphologic and structural features exist that warrant examination of a sectioned biopsy specimen. Recent studies indicate that CML is not a single entity and based on the findings of bone marrow biopsy sections the disease can be classified into two categories: granulocytic and mixed granulocytic-megakaryocytic types, according to the nature and predominance of the cellular proliferation. Sections may also reveal characteristic cellular proliferations of immature myeloid (haematopoietic) precursor cells adjacent to bony trabeculae (paratrabecular accumulation of blast cells). The extent of such infiltrations may also help predict the transformation of CML into an acute blastic phase.

Hairy Cell Leukaemia (HCL)

In this malignancy a bone marrow biopsy is usually diagnostic and presents a typical picture. It shows the characteristic cytologic features of hairy cells (round, oval, or kidney shaped nuclei whose chromatin, unlike that of small lymphocytes, shows little clumping). Unlike CLL and other lymphoid infiltrations of the marrow, hairy cells are loosely arranged, widely separated (an appearance probably due to their large cytoplasmic volume) and are enmeshed in a reticulin network which also contains plasma and mast cells and numerous free erythrocytes. Bone marrow aspiration is usually difficult due to presence of marrow fibrosis and as a result it yields either an unsatisfactory specimen or a dry tap.

Multiple myeloma (MM)

This haematologic malignancy is characterised by multifocal neoplastic proliferations of plasma cells. Bone marrow examination still remains the cornerstone in establishing the diagnosis. In classic cases, the morphologic diagnosis of MM is straightforward and not difficult. In such cases the bone marrow aspirate and/or biopsy sections show the presence of large clusters or infiltrates of plasma cells (mature, intermediate, immature or plasmablastic type) that replace the normal haematopoeitic elements. However, in other cases the diagnosis can be extremely difficult. This may be due to several reasons. First, the plasma cell infiltration may be associated with significant marrow fibrosis. The marrow aspiration in these cases is often very difficult and results in an unsatisfactory (nondiagnostic) sample, whereas a bone marrow biopsy section may prove to be diagnostic in this situation. Second, because of the multifocal nature of the disease process a bone marrow aspirate may fail to provide a diagnostic specimen; in such instances there is a greater likelihood, that a bone marrow biopsy will provide the required atypical tissue for diagnosis. Further, because sectioned specimens offer an insight into the undisturbed distribution of bone marrow cells, such preparations are more likely to permit the recognition of (normal) perivascular location of plasma cells versus the irregular distribution of pathologic proliferations. Thirdly, in cases where the bone marrow aspirate and/or section contain abnormal cells that cannot be definitely identified as belonging to the plasma cell series, it may still be possible to reveal their plasmacytic identity through the immunoperoxidase staining of plastic embedded bone marrow biopsy sections.

Hodgkin's Disease (HD)

Although the importance of bone marrow biopsy in the diagnosis and management of patients with Hodgkin's disease (HD) has been debated, they are still conducted in most centers as the detection of marrow involvement not only affects the level of pathologic staging but also influences the approach to therapy. In addition, a positive marrow biopsy obviates the need for a staging laparotomy. Although the incidence of bone marrow involvement in HD (as reported in the literature) varies considerably (2–32%), in a significant number of cases, typical Reed-Sternberg cells or their mononuclear variant can be identified in marrow sections. The extent of marrow involvement in a given bone marrow biopsy can vary from small focal lesions to almost complete replacement of the marrow.

Of the patients that do demonstrate medullary infiltration the pattern of involvement in the section is diffuse in 70-80% of the cases and focal in the remainder. In some studies marrow involvement has been shown to be one of the most important factors in predicting an unfavourable course of the disease. Nevertheless it has also been shown that in a large majority of cases with negative biopsies various nonspecific alterations were present in the marrow. These findings had predictive value: hypoplasia, exudative and leukaemoid reactions indicated a poor prognosis, while epithelioid cell granulomas and lymphocytic aggregates constituted more favourable signs.

Non-Hodgkin's Lymphoma (NHL)

A bone marrow examination is now considered an integral part of the initial diagnosis and staging of patients with non-Hodgkin's lymphoma. Bone marrow (core) biopsies are essential for this as aspirates have a high incidence of false negatives. Bilateral biopsies are generally believed to be superior to unilateral biopsies because the increased volume of marrow that is obtained enhances the likelyhood of finding a focal lesion. Some benefits are also derived from examining tissues obtained from two anatomically distant sites. Bone marrow biopsies are useful for evaluating patients' responses to chemotherapy and for following previously treated patients for evidence of recurrent disease.

Bone Disease

Bone marrow biopsies are critical for histomorphometric analysis of metabolic and non-metabolic bone disorders which are characterised by alterations in the amount and structure of cortical and trabecular bone; the amount, extent, and width of osteoid seams; and the extent of osteoclastic resorption surfaces. The abnormalities of bone formation, resorption and mineralization (osteoporosis, osteomalacia, osteodystrophy, Paget's disease etc.) may be diagnosed by bone marrow biopsy long before their effects are evident on X-ray films. For the performance of bone histomorphometry undecalcified bone marrow biopsy sections are essential because of the conservation of the differences between calcified and uncalcified bone (osteoid) which is required for the recognition of bone abnormalities.

Non-haematologic Malignancies

Documentation of the presence or absence of metastases to the skeletal system is an important step in the evaluation of the patient with a malignancy. It has long been appreciated that the red, well-vascularised haematopoietic marrow is one of the sites most commonly involved with matastases of non-haematologic malignancies (solid tumours). In patients with cancer of the breast or prostate, as well as those with neuroblastoma and small cell carcinoma of the lung, metastatic disease is initially documented in the marrow more frequently than in any other site. It is unfortunate that marrow biopsies are not routinely performed on most patients with solid tumours. It has been reported, for example, that patients with evidence of metastatic carcinoma of the breast in the marrow had a significantly higher relapse rate than did patients whose marrow did not have this manifestation. Clearly the demonstration of bone marrow metastasis in such patients will profoundly influence the choice of the therapeutic approach.

Marrow infiltrated with tumour tissue, including malignant lymphoma, can be difficult to aspirate and consequently a dry tap occurs relatively frequently. The sensitivity of histologic diagnosis of breast cancer from bone marrow (core) biopsies when compared with that obtained from aspirates or clot sections, was found to be superior; however, maximal success was obtained when both the biopsy and the aspirate were examined. Bilateral bone marrow biopsies are perhaps more sensitive in this regard because of the larger volume of tissue and the fact that two sites are examined.

NEWER DEVELOPMENTS AND FUTURE DIRECTIONS

The development and application of enzymatic and immunological techniques (e.g. immunoperoxidase) to decalcified (paraffin-embedded) and undecalcified (plastic-embedded) bone marrow biopsy sections continues to improve the haematologist's diagnostic capabilities. The use of monoclonal antibodies that react selectively with normal and abnormal haematopoietic cells as well as metastatic tumour cells in the marrow has further improved the diagnostic possibilities. In addition, the molecular genetic techniques, such as *in situ* mRNA hybridisation, interphase cytogenetics and PCR amplification of DNA for evaluation of minimal residual leukaemia/lymphoma in bone marrow biopsies are opening new frontiers in the etiologic and diagnostic evaluation of bone marrow biopsies in various haematologic and non-haematologic malignant conditions.

SELECTED READING

Beckstead, J.H. and Bainton, D. (1980) Enzyme histochemistry on bone marrow biopsies: reactions useful in the differential diagnosis of leukemia and lymphoma applied to 2-micron plastic sections. *Blood*, **55**, 386–394.

Bierman, H.R. and Kelly, K.H. (1956) Multiple marrow aspiration in man from the posterior ilium. *Blood*, **11**, 370–374.

Block, M. (1979) Text atlas of Hematology. Philadelphia; Lea and Febiger.

Brunning, R.D., Bloomfield., C.D., McKenna, R.W. *et al.* (1975) Bilateral trephine bone marrow biopsies in lymphoma and other neoplastic diseases. *Ann. Intern. Med.*, **82**, 365–366.

Burkhardt, R. (1971) Bone marrow and bone tissue: Color atlas of clinical histopathology. Berlin: Springer-Verlag.

Burkhardt, R., Frisch, B. and Bartl, R. (1982) Bone marrow biopsy in haematological disorders. *J. Clin. Pathol.*, **35**, 257–284.

Burkhardt, R. (1956) Myelotomy, a new method for combined cytohistology of bone marrow biopsy. *Blut*, **2**, 267–276.

Buss. D.H., Prichard, R.W., Hartz, J.W. *et al.* (1987) Comparison of the usefulness of bone marrow sections and smears in diagnosis of multiple myeloma. *Haematol. Pathol.*, **1**, 35–43.

Ehret, W., Schlag, R. and Burkhard, R. (1981) The causative and prognostical bearing on the aplastic syndrome of inflammatory bone marrow changes. Sixth meeting of International Society of Haematology, European and African Division, Athens, Greece, August 30 – September 4.

Ellis, L.D., Jensen, W.N. and Westerman, M.P. (1964) Needle biopsy of bone and marrow. *Arch. Intern. Med.*, **114**, 213–221.

Fey, M.F., Theilkas, L. and Tobler, A. (1990) Bone marrow trephine biopsies as a source of nucleic acids for molecular diagnosis of haematological neoplasms. *Br. J. Haematol.*, **74**, 229–231.

Frisch, B and Bartl, R. (1990) Atlas of bone marrow pathology: Current Histopathology Series (ed) G.A. Gresham, Kluwer Academic Publishers, Dordrecht.

Frisch. B., Bartl, R. and Burkhardt, R. (1982) Bone marrow biopsy in clinical medicine:and overview. *Haematologia*, **3**, 245–285.

Georgii, A., Vykoupil, K.F. and Thiele. J. (1984) Classification of chronic myeloproliferative diseases by bone marrow biopsies. Haematological and cytogenetic findings and clinical course. *Bibl. Haematol.*, **50**, 41–56.

Ghedini, G. (1908) Studi sulla patologia del midollo osseo umano vivente. I. Punctura explorative tecnica. *Clin. Med. Ital.*, **47**, 724–???.

Hodges, E., Stacy, G., White, D. *et al.* (1991) Histologic, immunophenotypic and genotypic analyses of bone marrow trephines from patients with non-Hodgkin's lymphoma. *Leuk. Res.*, **15**, 1117–1124.

Hutt, M.S.R., Smith, P., Clark, A.E. and Pinniger, J.L. (1952) The value of rib biopsy in the study of marrow disorders. *J. Clin. Pathol.*, **5**, 246–249.

Islam, A., Archimbaud, A., Henderson, E.S. and Han, T. (1988) Glycol methacrylate embedding for light microscopy II. Immunohistochemistry on semi-thin sections of undecalcified marrow core. *J. Clin. Pathol.*, **41**, 892–896.

Islam, A. (1982) A new bone marrow biopsy needle with core securing device. *J. Clin. Pathol.*, **35**, 359–366.

Islam, A. and Frisch, B. (1985) Plastic embedding in routine histology:1. Section preparation from undecalcified marrow core. *Histopathology*, **9**, 1263–1276.

Islam, A. and Henderson, E.S. (1987) Glycol methacrylate embedding for light microscopy. 1. Enzyme histochemistry on sections of undecalcified marrow core. *J. Clin. Pathol.*, **40**, 1194–1200.

Islam, A. and Henderson, E.S. (1990) The role of bone marrow biopsy in haematological disorders with special reference to plastic embedded material. *Haematol. Rev.*, **4**, 1–12.

Islam, A., Catovsky, D., Goldman, G.M. and Galton, D.A.G. (1979) Value of long core biopsy in detection of discrete bone marrow lesions. *Lancet*, **i**, 878.

Islam, A. (1988). Value of long core biopsy in the detection of discrete bone marrow lesions. *Histopathology*, **12**, 641–648.

Islam, A. (1983). A new bone marrow aspiration needle to overcome the sampling errors inherent in the technique of bone marrow aspiration. *J. Clin. Pathol.*, **36**, 954–958.

Islam, A. (1991) Value of plastic embedded bone marrow biopsy in the detection of residual disease and prediction of outcome of therapy in patients with acute myeloid leukemia. *Hematol. Rev.*, **5**, 129–140.

Islam, A. (1993) Proposal for a classification of acute myeloid leukaemia based on plastic embedded bone marrow biopsy sections. *Leuk. Res.*, **17**, 421–427.

Islam, A., Catovsky, D., Goldman, J.M. and Galton, D.A.G. (1984) Studies on cellular interactions between stromal and haemopoietic stem cells in normal and leukaemic bone marrows. *Bibl. Haematol.*, **50**, 17–30.

Islam, A., Catovsky, D., Goldman, J.M. and Galton, D.A.G. (1985) Bone marrow biopsy changes in acute myeloid leukaemia. 1. Observations before chemotherapy. *Histopathology*, **9**, 939–957.

Islam, A., Glomski, C. and Henderson, E.S. (1990). Bone lining (endosteal) cells and hematopoiesis: a light microscopic study of normal and pathologic human bone marrow. *Anatomical Record.*, **227**, 300–306.

Islam, A. (1992) The origin and spread of human leukemia. *Medical Hypothesis*, **39**, 110–118.

Islam, A., Catovsky D. and Galton, D.A.G. (1980) Histological study of bone marrow regeneration following chemotherapy for acute myeloid leukaemia and chronic granulocytic leukaemia in blast transformation. *Br. J. Haematol.*, **45**, 535–540.

Islam, A. and Henderson. E.S. (1988) Prediction of impending blast cell transformation in chronic granulocytic leukemia. *Histopathology*, **12**, 633–639.

Jacob, P. (1995) Choice of needle for bone marrow trephine biopsies. *Haematol. Rev.*, **9**, 163–168.

James, L.P., Stass, S.A. and Schumacher, H.R. (1980) Value of imprint preparations of bone marrow biopsies in hematologic diagnosis. *Cancer*, **46**, 173–177.

Jamshidi, K., Windschitl, H.E. and Swaim, W.R. (1971) A new biopsy needle for bone marrow. *Scand J. Haematol.*, **8**, 69–72.

Knowles, S. and Hoffbrand, A.V. (1980) Bone marrow aspiration and biopsy. *Br. Med. J.*, **281**, 204-205.

Krause, J.R. (1983) An appraisal of the value of the bone marrow biopsy in the assesment of proliferative lesions of the bone marrow. *Histopathology*, **7**, 627–644.

Landys, K and Stenram, S. (1975) Bone marrow biopsy of the posterior iliac crest with Gidlund's instrument in malignant diseases. *Scand. J. Haematol.*, **15**, 104–108.

Laughln, M., Islam, A., Barcos, M., Meade, P. *et al.* (1988) Bone marrow fibrotic changes in hairy cell leukemia in response to alpha interferon therapy. *Blood*, **72**, 936–939.

MacIntyre, E.A., Hudson, B.W., Linch, D.C. *et al.* (1987) The value of staging bone marrow trephine biopsy in Hodgkin's disease. *Euro. J. Haematol.*, **39**, 66–70.

Maschek H, Gutzmer, R., Choritz, H. and Georgii, A. (1995) Comparison of scoring systems in primary myelodysplastic syndromes. *Ann. Hematol.*, **70**, 301–308.

McFarland, W. and Dameshek, W. (1958) Biopsy of bone marrow with the Vim-Silverman Needle. *J.A.M.A.*, **166**, 1464–1466.

McKenna, R.W., and Hernandez, J.A. (1988) Bone marrow in malignant lymphoma. In: *Haematology Oncology Clinics of North America*, Ed. B.H. Hyun, **2**, 617–635.

Peabody, F.W. (1927) Pathology of bone marrow in pernicious anemia. *Am. J. Pathol.*, **3**, 179–202.

Podzimek, K., Kerekes, Z., Chrobak, L. *et al.* (1994) The value of bone marrow biopsy in the prognosis of hairy cell leukemia (HCL). *Neoplasma.*, **41**, 325–330.

Rozman, C., Hernandez-Nieto, L., Montserrat, E. and Brugues, R. (1981) Prognostic significance of bone marrow patterns in chronic lymphocytic leukaemia. *Br. J. Haematol.*, **47**, 529–537.

Rywlin, A.M. (1976) Histopathology of the bone marrow. Little, Brown and Company, Boston

Shpall, E..J., Gee, A.P., Hogan, C. *et al.* (1996) Bone marrow metastases in *Hematology/ Oncology Clinics of North America*. Hematologic Complications of Cancer. Eds. S.D. Nimer and D.W. Golde. Vol 10 (2), April 1996.

Te Velde, J. and Haak, H.L. (1979) Histology of bone marrow failure, a follow-up study in aplastic anaemia. In: H. Heimpel, E.C. Gordon-Smith, B. Kubanek, eds. Aplastic anemia: pathophysiology and approaches to therapy. Berlin, Heidelberg, New York, Springer-Verlag, **24**, 15–25.

Tricot, G., De Wolf, P.C., Vlietinck, R. *et al.* (1984) Bone marrow histology in myelodysplastic syndrome: II. Prognostic value of abnormal localization of immature precursors in MDS. *Br. J. Haematol.*, **58**, 217–225.

Turkel, H. and Bethell, F.H. (1943) Biopsy of bone marrow performed by a new and simple instrument. *J. Lab. Clin. Med.*, **28**, 1246–1250.

Hyun, B.H. (editor) Hematology/Oncology Clinics of North America, Vol 2 (4), December 1988.

Oppedal, B.R., Storm-Mathisen, I., Kemshead, J.T. *et al.* (1989) Bone marrow examination in neuroblastoma patients: A morphologic, immunocytochemical, and immunohistochemical study. *Hum Pathol.*, **20**, 800–805.

INDEX